FROM
MOUNTAIN
TO
METROPOLIS

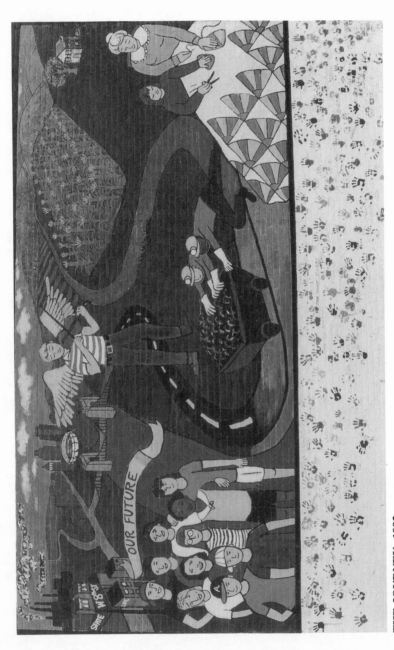

THE JOURNEY, 1993

A 26 by 16 foot mural painted by teenagers in Lower Price Hill, one of Cincinnati's Appalachian neighborhoods.

Photo: Matthew Obermiller

FROM MOUNTAIN TO METROPOLIS

Appalachian Migrants in American Cities

Edited by
Kathryn M. Borman
and
Phillip J. Obermiller

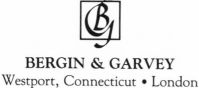

BERGIN & GARVEY
Westport, Connecticut • London

Library of Congress Cataloging-in-Publication Data

From mountain to metropolis : Appalachian migrants in American cities
    / edited by Kathryn M. Borman and Phillip J. Obermiller.
        p.   cm.
    Includes bibliographical references and index.
    ISBN 0-89789-367-0 (alk. paper)
    1. Appalachian Region, Southern. 2. Mountain whites (Southern
States). 3. Rural-urban migration—Southern States. I. Borman,
Kathryn M. II. Obermiller, Phillip J.
    F217.A65F76   1994
    974—dc20   93-11855

British Library Cataloguing in Publication Data is available.

Library of Congress Catalog Card Number: 93-11855
ISBN: 0-89789-367-0

First published in 1994

Bergin & Garvey, 88 Post Road West, Westport, CT 06881
An imprint of Greenwood Publishing Group, Inc.

Printed in the United States of America

The paper used in this book complies with the
Permanent Paper Standard issued by the National
Information Standards Organization (Z39.48-1984).

10 9 8 7 6 5 4 3 2 1

To Louise Spiegel and Stuart Faber,
abiding friends of urban Appalachians

Contents

II. HEALTH AND ENVIRONMENTAL ISSUES

III. SOCIAL AND EDUCATIONAL ISSUES

Illustrations

Introduction

This is a book about migration and its consequences. It is not about traversing oceans or international borders but about crossing real boundaries in one's own country. Internal migration is occurring today in every part of the world and on a massive scale. Families are leaving the mountainous hinterlands of Peru and China and Mexico for Lima and Shanghai and Mexico City. The same phenomenon is taking place in Africa and India.

More highly developed countries are not exempt from this trend. Since World War II, many farm laborers have moved from Italy's Mezzogiorno into the industrialized cities of the north in search of jobs. Thousands of fishermen and their families left the Canadian Maritime Provinces for the factories of Ontario and the shops of Toronto. In the United States, Appalachian miners left the coal towns of their mountain region for the car towns in Michigan, Ohio, Indiana, and Illinois.

These migrants are natives in their own countries: they speak the same languages, worship the same deities, and share the same culture as their compatriots. Yet they are different: their speech shows traces of a dialect or a regional accent, their religious beliefs focus on the fundamentals, and their folkways differ considerably from those of the receiving population. The new arrivals come in search of economic assimilation but are not necessarily eager to be socialized into the norms and customs of the dominant urban culture.

The differences go well beyond the simplistic dichotomy between rural and urban lifestyles. Most people living in Appalachia today have immediate satellite access to the best and the worst of mainstream American culture. If they should decide to experience it outside their living rooms, many are only a few hours' drive from a major metropolitan area. Yet they do not necessarily want to adopt the elements of an urban lifestyle as their own. They operate from a set of values that are at least different in degree, a difference that many Appalachian people find worth keeping and protecting. Appalachian migrants to urban and suburban areas behave similarly, accepting and integrating what they find valuable in the urban milieu and resisting the rest.

This volume focuses on Appalachians as a case study of internal migration in developed countries. As with many other internal migrant groups, Appalachian migration began before World War II and peaked in the decade following. It has not stopped since that time and often parallels national economic conditions: flows of outmigration are heavy in times of economic expansion, and return migration occurs in recessionary times. Back-and-forth (shuttle) migration occurs constantly as rural residents of the region explore for new economic opportunities or as urban Appalachians enjoy a period of cultural refreshment in the mountains.

Today millions of Appalachians are living in cities across the United States, often in urban enclaves that include people several generations removed from the migration experience. Assimilation has claimed some of the migrants' children and grandchildren; they no longer regard themselves, or are regarded by others, as Appalachian or "from the mountains."

Many urban Appalachians, however, have maintained their cultural ties to the region and its values. This group has been characterized as an "emergent" ethnic group. Many urban Appalachians have borne the burden of discrimination and often carry the stigma of "hillbilly" in their communities, schools, and places of work.

As internal migrants, Appalachians have experienced several stages in the process of settling into their new urban neighborhoods. The earliest urban categorization of Appalachian newcomers was obviously that of "migrant." Transience was the operative concept for interpreting Appalachian behavior in the first stage after migration. Adults were viewed as mobile and undependable because of job absenteeism related to visits "back home"; the same reason lay behind the stigmatizing label of "chronic truant" applied to Appalachian students. The image of instability was reinforced by frequent changes of address within and among port-of-entry neighborhoods as the newcomers sought decent jobs and housing. As a result of this early perception of Appalachian migrants as transients, they were viewed initially as a temporary problem that eventually would be resolved through return migration.

In the second stage following migration, the influx of Appalachians was interpreted more realistically. The spreading realization that large numbers of the migrants were becoming permanent residents gave rise to a new interpretation of their presence: Appalachians were no longer regarded primarily as transients but now were viewed as an abiding social problem; this perception was heightened by the social welfare activism of the 1960s inspired by Great Society programs such as Volunteers in Service to America (VISTA) and Model Cities.

The social problem approach to internal migration has three major drawbacks. First, it seems to imply that those who experience a problem need merely to adjust their own behavior in order to overcome their difficulties. According to this mode of thought, it is the migrant's responsibility to accommodate to the dominant culture. Second, focusing on the problem does not necessarily bring the solution any closer. Hiring more substance abuse counselors, for instance, may not lower the rate of substance abuse; putting more child welfare workers on the streets may result in increased reporting of child abuse but may not stop the incidence. The third limitation of the social problem approach is that defining urban Appalachians as only, or even primarily, uneducated residents of poor neighborhoods is simply inaccurate. It is more accurate to balance the reality of grinding inner-city poverty with the reality of stable Appalachian families living in working-class neighborhoods scattered across the metropolitan area. In short, too narrow a focus on the social problem approach contributes to a blindness to the structural problems that many urban Appalachians face.

As successful advocacy and service organizations arose in urban Appalachian neighborhoods, a third stage of Appalachian identity began to emerge. In addition to a legitimate concern for ameliorating the social problems faced by urban Appalachians, the idea of Appalachians as a social group was promoted actively. In the late 1970s, a new movement began to establish an ethnic identity for urban Appalachians. Several factors were involved in this development. The first was the ethnic revival that was taking place among immigrant groups across the nation; "Appalachian ethnicity" became a fashionable substitute phrase for "Appalachian identity." Second, as a result of the black pride movement, cultural distinctiveness became an acceptable basis for developing special programs supported by government and private philanthropy. The third advantage in using the concept of ethnicity was its long-standing acceptance in the social sciences. The movement from migration to ethnic group formation and finally to the process of assimilation was a well-established dynamic in the history of white immigrant groups in the United States. Ethnicity inevitably points to assimilation, an idealistic, if inaccurate, outcome cherished in our national value system.

The fourth stage following migration might be considered in terms of social ecology. By definition, our understanding of Appalachia is ecological; therefore, so is our understanding of who is Appalachian. The ecological definition implies some vague cultural "content" in the definition of *Appalachian*. In contrast, the concept of Appalachians as a social problem depends heavily on the notion of Appalachians as having definite cultural characteristics that are dysfunctional in the contemporary urban milieu. Similarly, the social group perspective assumes the existence of a distinctive Appalachian culture, although it takes a more positive and more prideful approach.

The ecological definition of urban Appalachians has taken on a new importance as the migration experience fades. It is increasingly difficult to identify urban Appalachians with reference to their migration. Consequently, they are defined through knowledge of their demographic characteristics and settlement patterns. The ecological definition of Appalachians in cities depends on their neighborhood of residence rather than on their participation in or relationship to the migration experience. Interestingly, the ecological model tends to favor social class factors over cultural characteristics in the identification of Appalachians.

Urban Appalachians were viewed in the urban setting first as transients and later as having a complex set of social problems that needed remediating. As the Appalachian community gained control of its own image in the 1970s, a new ethnic identity was promoted, that of urban Appalachians. As the migration experience fades further into the background, it is reasonable to expect that the social class status of urban Appalachians will receive more emphasis.

To date, the literature on urban Appalachians has focused on the first three stages described above. *The Invisible Minority*, edited by Philliber and McCoy (1981), emphasizes the social problem aspects of Appalachian migration: issues surrounding migration, discrimination and stereotyping, jobs, and housing. Philliber's *Appalachian Migrants in Urban America* (1981b) deals explicitly with the stage of ethnic group formation. *Too Few Tomorrows*, edited by Obermiller and Philliber (1987), covers topics in both the social problem stage and the social group stage.

The current volume looks beyond the earlier stages of migration to its social consequences. Many urban Appalachians have settled into their jobs, their housing, and their identity. Yet as this migrant population has matured into several generations of urban Appalachians, new issues have arisen: acquiring an education, gaining access to health care systems, and preserving cultural values.

Part I provides an overview of current migration patterns, recent demographic information, and the cultural perseverance to be found among urban Appalachians. Chapter 1 examines the current demographic status of two generations of Appalachian migrants, while Chapter 2 contrasts the "settling in" patterns of Appalachian migrants in two metropolitan areas, Cincinnati and Pittsburgh. Chapter 3 shows the endurance of specific cultural behaviors across generations by examining where and how urban Appalachians are buried. The outcomes of migration for Appalachian women are studied in Chapter 4.

In Part II, devoted to health care and environmental concerns, each chapter uses the comparative method to show the differences as well as the similarities between urban blacks and Appalachians. Chapter 5 focuses on health care needs by taking the consumer's perspective. Chapter 6 highlights the different strategies used by urban Appalachians and urban blacks to obtain information about health care, whereas Chapter 7 is devoted to the health status of urban Appalachian children. Chapter 8 considers attitudes and opinions regarding the environment shared by Appalachians and other urban groups.

Part III focuses on issues concerning the education of urban Appalachian children, particularly those whose economic situation and residential location have marginalized them. Chapter 9 considers strategies for assessing students' needs and constructing intervention strategies in a manner that is ethnically valid. Chapter 10 considers specific cross-cultural interactional patterns that are utilized by the authors in serving their urban Appalachian clients requiring special education services. The issues raised by participants in a youth program designed to meet their particular needs are addressed in Chapter 11. Adult workers in a company-based literacy program express their fears, concerns, and desires for adequate skills in reading and writing in Chapter 12. Chapter 13 considers issues related to the social organization of schools and schooling for urban Appalachian children that are frequently neglected by those who are unfamiliar with Appalachian culture. Finally, Chapter 14 raises concerns about the nature of community-based research in the cities where Appalachians live.

This volume, overall, presents new ways of characterizing the work of social service providers in Appalachian neighborhoods. Each of the authors in this volume are committed as activists and advocates to urge service providers and researchers to ground themselves thoroughly in urban Appalachian settings as they carry out their work.

PJO
KMB

Cincinnati

I

Migration Patterns, Demographics, and Cultural Perseverance

1

Living City, Feeling Country: The Current Status and Future Prospects of Urban Appalachians

Phillip J. Obermiller and Michael E. Maloney

The term *urban Appalachian* was coined in the early 1970s by Appalachians living in midwestern cities to describe themselves after realizing that *Appalachian migrant* was no longer appropriate. Most of them were not migrants in the sense of having moved recently from one region to another, or in the sense that applies to migrant farm workers.

Urban Appalachian became the favored term to describe those people and their descendants who had come from the Appalachian region to live and work in cities outside Appalachia. The original migrants are referred to as first-generation migrants; their children, as second-generation migrants; their grandchildren, as third-generation; and so on. The term *urban Appalachian* also is used at times to characterize the population of urban centers within Appalachia such as Knoxville or Pittsburgh, but this usage is less frequent.

As used in this chapter, *urban Appalachian* includes both migrants to cities outside the Appalachian region and their descendants of whatever generation. For simplicity, we will refer to the first and second generations as the *early generations* and to the third, fourth, and following generations as the *subsequent generations*.

Most urban Appalachians now have lived outside the region for all or most of their lives. Because millions of Appalachians have made the transition from rural newcomers to long-term residents of urban neighborhoods, new questions are being asked. More than three decades have passed since the peak years of Appalachian migration. How are these people and their children faring in the cities? How do they compare with other urban groups on key social indicators? Are Appalachians assimilating into urban culture or returning to the region? What are some of the key social policy questions they have raised for urban administrators and politicians?

In this chapter, we will attempt to shed some light on these questions. To do so, we must draw on various studies that use a variety of methods. The Cincinnati metropolitan area has an extensive history of Appalachian immigration and an equally extensive collection of current social research on urban Appalachians. Although these studies focus on Appalachians in the urban counties of northern Kentucky and southwestern Ohio, we believe that the findings can be extrapolated to urban Appalachians living in similar metropolitan areas outside the region.

We will proceed by first discussing the demographic information we have on first- and second-generation urban Appalachians. Then we consider the conditions affecting the subsequent generations. We conclude with an analysis of the issues that will affect urban Appalachians in the 1990s.

THE EARLY GENERATIONS: A DEMOGRAPHIC PROFILE

In both 1980 and 1989, the Greater Cincinnati Survey included questions that allowed for identification of first- and second-generation urban Appalachians. The surveys used a random-digit dialing technique to contact approximately 1,000 respondents in Hamilton County, Ohio, in which Cincinnati is located. The sampling procedure and the response rate allowed for confidence intervals ranging between 3 and 5 percent for each question. The respondents were divided into three comparison groups: white non-Appalachians ("white"), black non-Appalachians ("black"), and white Appalachians ("Appalachian"). Because of their relatively small size in the sample (2.3%) and their ambiguous status, black Appalachians were not included in either the black or the Appalachian cohort (see Philliber and Obermiller 1987).

The early generations of urban Appalachians make up a substantial portion of the Hamilton County population. In 1980 they constituted one quarter of the people living in the county: nine years later they still accounted for one in five of the county's residents. Although migration has slowed, natural increase is adding to the urban Appalachian cohort; when we take the third and fourth generations into consideration, we estimate that Appalachians may account for as much as 40 percent of the county's total population.

First- and second-generation urban Appalachians are divided about evenly in cohort size, but (as one would expect) the age dynamics differ. The average age of first-generation Appalachians in 1989 was 49; the average age for the second generation was 43.

Although the longitudinal data show that Appalachians are aging faster than non-Appalachians and that the first generation is aging more slowly than the second generation, we must be cautious in interpreting these figures. First of all, our sample is composed of only the first two generations of Appalachians; therefore, the Appalachians appear to be older than the non-Appalachian cohort because the latter does not select out particular generations for analysis. Second, because first-generation Appalachians naturally have a higher mortality rate than the second generation, their average age appears to be rising more slowly over time.

Despite these cautions, the data show clearly that first- and second-generation Appalachians form a large cohort whose average age is substantially above that of the non-Appalachian groups in Hamilton County. In 1989 the average age of blacks was 39; for whites, it was 43; and for Appalachians, it was 46. The early migrants and their children are growing old, and this fact will have a strong effect on the interpretation of the other Appalachian demographic characteristics.

The ratio of men to women in the urban Appalachian community is shifting over time to a higher proportion of women. By 1989, 61 percent of the Appalachians surveyed were women, and 39 percent were men. This finding is consistent with an aging population in which men tend to die at an earlier age than women.

The fact that migration has slowed and that Appalachians are long-term residents in urban areas is documented in the 1989 figures on length of residence. For blacks the average length of residence in the county was 29 years; for whites, 32 years; and for Appalachians, 31. These figures represent a slight increase for blacks since 1980, a modest increase for whites, and a large increase for Appalachians. Again, this change can be linked to the age factor; because Appalachians tend to be older overall than the other groups, they have had a greater opportunity to establish a longer residency period. Nonetheless, we note that Appalachians are long-term urban residents with very few recent migrants among them; in 1989, only 3.5 percent had lived in the county 2 years or less, whereas 67.3 percent had lived there 21 years or more.

From another perspective on residency, Appalachians are becoming more urban over time. In 1980, 68.6 percent of the Appalachian respondents lived in the suburban areas of the county surrounding the city of Cincinnati; only 31.4 percent were city dwellers. By 1989 a significant shift had taken place: 44.4 percent lived in the city, and 55.6 percent lived elsewhere in the county. The comparative statistics show that the proportions of blacks and Appalachians living in the Cincinnati part of Hamilton County increased greatly in the period between 1980 and 1989. Cincinnati is becoming a city with a growing minority population that is mostly black and Appalachian.

The data on marital status and household size show that the urban Appalachian family remains a strong social unit. Appalachians are more likely to be married or widowed than either blacks or whites. Conversely, they are much less likely to have never married than either of the other two groups. More than 7 in 10 Appalachian respondents reported that they were married; this fact can be attributed in part to the higher average age of this group. This argument, however, is diminished somewhat by the fact that urban Appalachian divorce rates are about one third of those reported by blacks and on a par with those reported by whites.

The average household size for Appalachians (3.1) remained constant over the nine-year period between the two surveys and is about the same as that for blacks and whites. The average number of adults in Appalachian households (2.3) increased slightly from 1980 to 1989, while decreasing for the other two groups. The average number of children under age 18 in Appalachian households (0.77) declined between 1980 and 1989 and is lower than that of either blacks or whites. The larger number of adults and the smaller number of children in Appalachian households are consistent with the higher average age of the household members.

Urban Appalachians are the least likely of the three groups to report no religious affiliation. In 1989, 70 percent of those surveyed reported being Protestant, but nearly 20 percent reported being Catholic, a substantial gain in the latter category since 1980. The proportion of Protestants among Appalachians and blacks is similar; and these groups differ distinctly from the whites, half of whom are Catholic and two fifths of whom are Protestant.

Educational attainment improved for urban Appalachians in the interval between the two surveys. In 1989, Appalachians had fewer high school dropouts than in 1980 (17% vs. 27%) and more students in college or graduated from college (45% vs. 36%). In 1989, however, Appalachians held the same relative status in educational attainment as in 1980; that is, they fared better than blacks but worse than other whites. The data on educational attainment show that blacks are more likely to drop out of high school and college than Appalachians, whereas whites are more likely to complete high school and college than Appalachians. When the sample is confined to Appalachians living in inner-city neighborhoods, their educational outcomes are even worse than those for urban blacks (Obermiller and Oldendick 1989).

The overall occupational status of urban Appalachians declined between 1980 and 1989. During this period, Appalachians gained in the number of sales and clerical jobs they held (+14%), but lost ground in the categories of craftspersons (-10%) and operatives (-7%). Unfortunately, significant employment growth for Appalachians occurred in the lowest occupational category, that of laborers and service workers (+12%). Blacks also showed substantial growth in the labor and service category, although their growth in this area of employment was only half as large as for whites.

The unemployment rate among Appalachians declined slightly from 1980 to 1989 but was far more than twice the rates reported by both whites and blacks in the 1989 survey. This statistic, however, must be tempered with the knowledge that many Appalachians operate outside the standard employer/employee relationship; they work for themselves in the informal economy doing home maintenance, roofing, hauling, and appliance and auto repair; providing child care; and selling goods at flea markets. These people may not consider themselves as "employed" in the traditional sense, but they are working hard to maintain their family's income.

Between 1980 and 1989 the number of Appalachian families with total incomes of less than $20,000 a year declined, and the number with annual incomes greater than $30,000 a year rose. In the middle-income category ($20,000 to $30,000), however, Appalachian families lost ground. Overall the Appalachians' representation across the family income categories is on a par with that of whites and is significantly better than among black families. Although this pattern may differ from inner-city to suburban neighborhoods, it remained constant at the county level from 1980 to 1989. A significant portion of Appalachian family income is provided by women, four fifths of whom are in the labor force.

THE SUBSEQUENT GENERATIONS: PROSPECTS FOR THE FUTURE

The situation of subsequent generations of urban Appalachians can be described in more qualitative fashion. A minority have obtained a college education, have moved away from blue-collar Appalachian neighborhoods, and are largely assimilated into the larger urban culture. Others have moved from the old neighborhoods but maintain blue-collar lifestyles that include their extended family and a group of Appalachian friends as their primary social network. Most urban Appalachians, however, continue to live in working-class neighborhoods whose principal residents are other white Appalachians.

Appalachian neighborhoods vary greatly as to location within the metropolitan area and as to the residents' socioeconomic status. Some are inner-city neighborhoods characterized by multifamily rental units and high rates of underemployment, unemployment, and poverty. These communities are affected by the social problems typical of such areas: high rates of crime and delinquency, teen pregnancy, substance abuse, child neglect, and family violence. Although it is common to regard these neighborhoods as slums, it is more useful to view them as low-income ethnic neighborhoods or urban villages (Gans 1962). An urban village is an area of low-cost housing in which a group, usually immigrants, rebuilds the family, community, and economic structures that were debilitated by migration. Life in the urban village is more familiar to the earlier generations of Appalachian migrants than to the subsequent generations.

William Philliber (1981b) found that the majority of urban Appalachians in Cincinnati do not live in inner-city neighborhoods. Most live in working-class communities, some of which are located in the suburbs. Appalachians also make up a significant part of the population of small towns and cities that surround metropolitan core cities such as Cincinnati (Obermiller and Maloney 1990a).

Education is a critical issue for the Appalachians of the subsequent generations. Early migrants could obtain manufacturing jobs that merely required physical dexterity and some mechanical aptitude. Today, in an era when most jobs paying reasonable salaries require advanced skills, urban Appalachian students drop out of high school in large numbers (Maloney and Borman 1987). Many reasons have been advanced to explain the high rates of school failures and dropouts in this group (Maloney et al. 1989). School administrators point to absenteeism and to a lack of interest in education among Appalachian parents. Appalachians themselves regard urban public school systems as large, impersonal bureaucracies with little cultural sensitivity. Whatever the explanation, urban Appalachians in Ohio drop out of school at rates even higher than those of other cultural and racial minorities.

The early generations of Appalachians arrived in the cities during an era of industrial expansion and strong unions; semiskilled jobs were plentiful, wages were rising, and health and retirement benefits generally were available. Because of this blue-collar background, urban Appalachians of the subsequent generations have been devastated by the decline of the automobile, steel, and other manufacturing industries in the Midwest. These workers and their families have adapted in a variety of ways. Some have returned to the mountains, but this option is limited by the lack of work and housing in rural Appalachia. Others have moved to the urban growth centers of the South and the West in search of work. Some of those who stayed in the Midwest found replacement jobs in the industrial sector, but many have been forced to settle for lower-paying jobs in the service sector of the formal economy or to resort to work in the informal economy. Family income is maintained by increasing the number of workers; spouses and children all take jobs to supplement the household budget.

Appalachians still make heavy use of family networks to find employment or to obtain a temporary place to live while seeking a job. Those who lack family support may turn to public assistance or obtain help from their church or a local social agency, but this is considered a strategy of last resort. Appalachians living in inner-city areas who have lost the support of their families and of neighborhood social welfare agencies can be found living on the streets, sleeping in shelters for the homeless, and standing in the lines at soup kitchens.

Like education and employment, health conditions in the subsequent generations vary greatly. Urban Appalachians in poverty have high rates of coronary heart disease, diabetes, and work-related disabilities. Their children suffer from lack of perinatal care, poor nutrition, and the effects of urban pollution. Sexually transmitted diseases affect many Appalachian teenagers. Injuries related to work are common among all generations of urban Appalachians, as are illnesses due to stress and diet such as diabetes, hypertension, and heart disease (Obermiller and Oldendick 1989).

Are subsequent generations losing their Appalachian identity and assimilating into the cultural mainstream? Most urban Appalachians are concentrated in blue-collar enclaves in urban neighborhoods, in suburban communities, and in small towns. Because of their numbers they often form the majority population in these places. In addition to living near relatives and other people of Appalachian background, they associate with their own kind at work and in their churches, labor unions, civic associations, and schools, as well as in local bars and restaurants. Their music, dance, crafts, and artistic traditions are renewed constantly through arts and crafts festivals, bluegrass preservation societies, records, tapes, films, and radio programs. Although there are more Appalachians in Ohio's Miami Valley (Cincinnati, Hamilton, Middletown, Dayton, Xenia, Troy) than in all of eastern Kentucky, the residents of these cities make use of the easy access to their home places and kinfolk in the mountains. To a certain extent, urban Appalachians resemble Mexican-Americans in the southwestern United States who gain cultural support from visits or frequent communication with their home districts in rural Mexico.

Most studies of migrant groups find that ethnic identity begins to dwindle with the third generation (see Philliber 1987). The process of assimilation, however, is slowed by ethnic organizations with strong leadership, which promote the cultural heritage and the political concerns of the group. It is also hindered by the presence of discrimination and by the group's perception of exclusion from the economic and social mainstream. We believe that all of the factors we have cited are limiting the absorption of Appalachians into the dominant urban society. There is no danger that Appalachians will disappear from the social map of urban America in the 1990s.

COMMENTS AND POLICY RECOMMENDATIONS

We now turn to an analysis of data on urban Appalachians and a commentary on the social policy and program implications of this information. In discussing the data, we take care again to distinguish among urban Appalachians both by age (early generations vs. subsequent generations) and by socioeconomic status (suburban vs. inner-city).

The early generations of urban Appalachians are clearly an aging population. During the 1990s their concerns can be expected to move away from a focus on education and employment and toward health care. Moreover, many urban Appalachians are aging in place rather than returning to the region for retirement (Obermiller 1991). In fact, many elderly Appalachians are being moved from the region by their urban kinfolk to metropolitan areas, where health care facilities, nursing homes, retirement communities, and the potential for in-home care are much more abundant.

The aging of the early generations also has implications for urban Appalachian women, the traditional caregivers in their culture. At a time when the number of children per household is beginning to decline, and women's educational attainment and labor force participation have begun to increase, care for the elderly will become a larger part of the responsibilities in Appalachian households. Much of this duty will devolve upon the women.

From a policy standpoint, the aging of the urban Appalachian population will require more resources in health care and geriatric services. From a programmatic point of view, social welfare organizations must be concerned not only with the Appalachian elderly but also with their caregivers, most of whom will be working women.

Among the subsequent generations, adult education and job training will continue to be important issues. The longitudinal data show urban Appalachians losing ground on the socioeconomic treadmill; even as their educational attainment improves, the demand for education in the labor force increases at a higher rate. This fact explains why members of the early generations who increased their rates of high school completion are nonetheless slipping gradually into lower-status job categories. In these families, a stable income can be maintained only by maximizing the number of workers in the family. If the cost of living increases while family size remains stable, many working-class urban Appalachians will slip into poverty.

The situation for inner-city Appalachians is even more grim. Half of the adults in these neighborhoods have no more than a high school education, school dropout rates are as high as 75 percent, and youth unemployment is a serious problem. Although social problems persist in these neighborhoods, the urban Appalachian community is not without resources to deal with them. In Cincinnati, community schools have been founded to provide on-site General Equivalency Diploma (GED) programs, adult education courses, and college-level classes. As a social unit, the Appalachian extended family has been battered but not broken. It still provides the social and economic resources that enable its members to survive in the city.

Policymakers need to focus not only on the problems in the urban Appalachian community but also on the inherent strengths. They should make every effort to recognize and reinforce the successful survival mechanisms that are operating in low-income Appalachian neighborhoods. Academic and job training projects, for example, should be designed to bolster Appalachian family interaction and local community schooling initiatives. Social welfare programs should support local initiatives among urban Appalachians rather than attempting to supplant them.

School reform is a critical issue among urban Appalachians. In the inner-city school systems, stemming the dropout rates among Appalachian youths continues to be a concern for most of the community but for relatively few school administrators. In some suburban school systems the retention rates among Appalachian youths are better, but these students generally finish in the bottom half of their graduating class. One programmatic suggestion that has yet to be implemented widely is the inclusion of units on Appalachian studies in both teacher training sessions and school curricula.

Another area of concern implicit in the comparative survey data gathered in greater Cincinnati is the relationship between urban Appalachians, blacks, and whites. As we have noted, blacks and Appalachians are the two largest minorities in the city; yet non-Appalachian whites hold most of the economic and political power in Cincinnati. The black community is frustrated, fearing the loss of hard-won legislative and constitutional gains. Urban blacks are wary about sharing their meager power and resources with their Appalachian neighbors. Unless new means of cooperation are developed between these two groups, conflict over allocation of power and resources will increase.

The policy direction is clear: municipal governments in cities such as Cincinnati must hold mediation sessions with black and Appalachian leaders to discuss cooperation in conflict resolution and allocation of resources. Specific areas for mediation include control of community agencies and the allocation of employment and training funds. In education, black leaders favor school desegregation plans that entail districtwide busing, whereas urban Appalachians favor community control of neighborhood schools with local attendance. Resolution of these differences would allow both groups to focus on the quality of education they seek for their children.

Not all issues polarize urban blacks and Appalachians. For instance, both groups oppose police brutality and the displacement of low-income families from their neighborhoods. They share concerns about the inclusion of minority studies in school curricula and about the effects of heavy industrial pollution on their children (see Lower Price Hill Task Force 1990). Urban Appalachians and their black neighbors have great potential for either conflict or cooperation. The 1900s may well decide which approach will prevail.

CONCLUSION

In the next 10 years, urban Appalachians will continue to wrestle with the issues they have confronted in the past, particularly education and employment. Establishing cooperative relations with other racial or ethnic minorities will continue to be a priority in an era of shrinking resources. New concerns will include a stronger emphasis on health care for the elderly population and the very young. Adult education and job retraining will become increasingly important as the decade advances.

The urban Appalachians we have studied do not lack the resources necessary to deal with the changing urban scene. They are maintaining relatively strong family bonds, supporting and using their own cultural institutions and organizations, and devising new ways to deal with old problems. The future for urban Appalachians holds the promise of both great struggles and great successes.

2

Looking for Appalachians in Pittsburgh: Seeking Deliverance, Finding the Deer Hunter

Phillip J. Obermiller and Michael E. Maloney

Appalachia is an abiding symbol of rural white poverty in America. When the media need a visual clip, a sound bite, or a few column inches on rural poverty, reporters and photo journalists are dispatched to Appalachia. When presidential contenders need a social issue, their campaign trails often include a small Appalachian town as an opportune place for a quick speech and a few photos.

Apart from its symbolic function of invoking images of poverty, Appalachia remains fairly unknown to mainstream America. Millions of Appalachians, looking for work and seeking improved life chances for themselves and their families, have left the region and settled in metropolitan areas from Baltimore to Los Angeles. These migrants receive even less recognition than their kinfolk back in the mountains. Urban Appalachians have been characterized aptly as "the invisible minority"—invisible because their culture is not recognized and minority because when it is recognized, it is not accepted by individuals and institutions in the urban mainstream.

Appalachian migrants to cities such as Cincinnati have begun to organize, and they are imposing a severe strain on the assumptions, stereotypes, and biases of urban power brokers. Cincinnati's urban Appalachians are teaching government social service departments, philanthropic organizations, social welfare agencies, school systems, and mainline religious groups that ethnicity is not restricted to people of foreign lands and cultures, that poverty is not confined to urban blacks and rural whites, and that assimilation into the urban milieu is not a foregone conclusion for many rural-to-urban migrants.

In Pittsburgh the picture is entirely different. The city, the county (Allegheny), and all of western Pennsylvania lie within the Appalachian region as defined by the federal government, making the entire population of the Pittsburgh metropolitan area technically *Appalachian*. Yet there is no sign of an Appalachian cultural presence in Pittsburgh. Pittsburgh's history of immigration and its strong ethnic neighborhoods would lead most observers to believe that Appalachians are merely the most recent group of white ethnics to establish itself in the city. Yet Pittsburgh may be the only major metropolitan area in or near the Appalachian region without a significant Appalachian migrant population. This chapter explores the underlying reasons for this anomaly.

The authors, one Appalachian and the other of European ethnic stock, are familiar with the dynamics of Appalachian migration and ethnic neighborhood formation in Cincinnati and other midwestern cities. We traveled to Pittsburgh expecting to find hidden enclaves of "invisible" Appalachians. We visited several different neighborhoods in and around Pittsburgh, where we spoke with residents. We interviewed key informants across the city—preachers, social workers, educators, shopkeepers, university professors—and always asked where we might find a neighborhood populated by West Virginians or by "folks from the mountains." We scanned scholarly documents and daily newspapers, looking for hints of an Appalachian presence in Pittsburgh. Using annual county-to-county migration data produced jointly by the Census Bureau and the Internal Revenue Service, we studied migration flows out of Appalachia and into Allegheny County.

The results of our study are presented below as a comparison of two cities, Cincinnati and Pittsburgh. Cincinnati represents the 30 major metropolitan areas in which Appalachians can be found as a legitimate, if invisible, ethnic group. Pittsburgh, surrounded by Pennsylvania's Appalachian counties and readily accessible by Interstate 79 from West Virginia, stands alone; it represents the only known case in which Appalachian migration streams have almost entirely avoided an accessible industrial city.

The Appalachian region is composed of 399 counties, which lie across portions of Mississippi, Alabama, Georgia, Tennessee, South Carolina, North Carolina, Kentucky, Ohio, New York, Virginia, Maryland, nearly all of western Pennsylvania, and the entire state of West Virginia. Although Appalachians generally are perceived as a rural people, about 75 percent of the region's 1980 population lived in metropolitan or urban counties (Obermiller and Oldendick 1987). Major urban areas in the Appalachian region include Birmingham, Charleston, Chattanooga, Huntington, Huntsville, Knoxville, Pittsburgh, and Tuscaloosa. Cities located in counties bordering on the region include Atlanta, Buffalo, Cincinnati, and Memphis. Extractive industries, specifically coal mining, traditionally have formed the region's economic base; agriculture, forestry, tourism and recreation, and textile manufacturing are also components of the regional economy.

Significant cultural diversity exists in the Appalachian region. Eastern Ohio, for instance, contains areas of primarily Anglo-Saxon and Celtic background with historic links to Kentucky and Virginia. Other parts of the region were settled by people from New England and are not a part of the "upland south" cultural region. The river towns north of Marietta, Ohio, are home to large numbers of people with central and southern European heritages. Similar diversity is found in Appalachian Pennsylvania: Washington County appears to be influenced more strongly by the culture of the British Isles than are the steel towns along the Monongahela and Ohio rivers, where central European ethnicity is predominant.

What, then, do we mean when we say that a person is "Appalachian" or when we use terms such as *an Appalachian neighborhood*? Because *Appalachian* has such a variety of connotations and denotations, we will describe some of the most common usages and will state which one we are using at any given time. A politician might reasonably refer to all residents of the 399 counties in the region as Appalachian. This usage ignores the fact that many people living in the region may have moved there from other places, but many researchers employ this definition because of the availability of data. Researchers on Appalachian migration generally regard as Appalachian a person who was born in the region or whose forebears were born in the region. *Southern Appalachian* refers to people living in West Virginia and the mountainous areas south of there; *northern Appalachian* refers to people living in the hills of southeastern Ohio and in upland areas to the north.

Anthropologists studying value orientations go beyond these geographical and topographical distinctions; they define as Appalachian anyone who is tied to the region by ancestry and who shares the subcultural values of that area. Further distinctions could be made between mountain subcultures—for example, between farmers and miners, rural dwellers and small-town folk, or snake handlers and Primitive Baptists.

The Appalachians who migrated to metropolitan centers in large numbers, who clustered in blue-collar ethnic neighborhoods, and who experienced problems typical of most low-income migrants (underemployment, poverty, school failure, stereotyping, and discrimination) come primarily from the northern and southern Appalachian coalfields. As might be expected, this group is predominantly white, mostly Baptist or Pentecostal, and heavily blue-collar. They are mostly of Scots-Irish or

Anglo-Saxon heritage, speak with a distinct accent, and enjoy country and western, bluegrass, and old-time gospel music. When we went looking for Appalachians in Pittsburgh, these were the people we sought.

On the basis of these characteristics, we expected to find Appalachian neighborhoods filled with "hillbilly" bars and restaurants, Pentecostal and Baptist churches, and people speaking with mountaineer accents. Other typical lifestyle features of blue-collar Appalachian neighborhoods include pickup trucks equipped with hunting rifles, campers, body shops, and shade-tree mechanics working on their vehicles.

We acknowledge that there are other kinds of Appalachians in Pittsburgh—for example, professionals from West Virginia in suburban communities, blacks from eastern Kentucky in integrated middle-class neighborhoods, and blue-collar Poles and Italians from the mining counties of southwestern Pennsylvania in central city neighborhoods. Our point is not to deny Appalachian heritage to any of these groups but to recognize that they are quite likely to be highly assimilated into their new urban milieus not as Appalachians but as professional blacks or Poles or Italians.

A TALE OF TWO CITIES: CINCINNATI

Cincinnati's diversified industrial base is a key factor in its record of economic stability and balanced growth. Early immigrants from manufacturing cities in Germany established metal-casting foundries and precision machine tool companies that survive to this day. General Electric, one of the area's largest employers, fabricates and assembles precision parts for jet engines. Automobile companies such as Ford also employ many skilled workers in local plants.

Germans from more rural areas founded stockyards, abattoirs, and meat-packing plants that earned Cincinnati the sobriquet of "Porkopolis." These thrifty immigrants were famous for using "every part of the pig but the squeal," and their industrial legacy is equally as diverse: the Kroger meat and grocery chain, Procter & Gamble soap products, and Jergens cosmetics all have their headquarters in Cincinnati.

Following a pattern similar to that found in Pittsburgh, Cincinnati's early industrialists founded schools, philanthropic foundations, hospitals, banks, and insurance companies that provide a wide array of job possibilities. With its blend of employment opportunities in manufacturing, marketing, finance, health, and education, Cincinnati has long been a magnet for migrants in search of work.

Cincinnati is a city of strong neighborhood identities that convey more than a sense of location; they are also associated with specific ethnic and racial groups and with varying economic conditions. Historically, Cincinnati and its environs have been a major destination for Appalachian migrants. Between 1955 and 1960, the area ranked eighth among the receiving cities; nearly 1 of every 5 newcomer came from Appalachia. Between 1965 and 1970, 1 of every 10 recent migrants to the city was Appalachian (McCoy and Brown 1981). By 1981 greater Cincinnati ranked ninth among the 30 major receiving cities; nearly 1 of every 4 residents of the metropolitan area was either a first- or a second-generation Appalachian migrant (Obermiller and Oldendick 1987). Most Appalachian families came to Cincinnati to find jobs. They were generally young, married, less well educated than their urban counterparts, and frequently in the unskilled or semiskilled sector of the labor force. Many Appalachian workers found regular employment, joined unions, and became an integral part of the urban economy. Others, however, were less fortunate. Used by employers as a pool of surplus labor to augment the local labor force during cyclical busy seasons, these Appalachians became the working poor, who often slipped unnoticed into the urban underclass.

As an aggregate, first- and second-generation Appalachians are not doing badly. When compared with non-Appalachian whites and non-Appalachian blacks in the Cincinnati metropolitan area, white Appalachians have a socioeconomic status lower than that of the other whites but higher than that of the blacks. As for schooling, work, and income, white Appalachians are faring better than blacks but less well than their other white counterparts.

A different picture emerges, however, when the metropolitan Appalachian population is divided between residents of Cincinnati and residents of the suburbs. About half of the Appalachian population lives within the city limits of Cincinnati, and members of this group fall consistently below their suburban counterparts on a variety of economic and social indicators: they are younger, are less well educated, earn less income, work at less prestigious jobs, and are more likely to be living alone (Community Chest and Council of the Cincinnati Area 1983; Philliber 1981b).

When Appalachians living in the city of Cincinnati are contrasted with their non-Appalachian black and white counterparts, their situation appears even poorer. The three indicators of socioeconomic status—education, occupation, and income—show the non-Appalachian whites to be at the higher end of the scale, the white Appalachians at the lower end, and the blacks in the middle. Only 32 percent of the non-

Appalachian whites have less than a high school education, for example, but this proportion rises to 47 percent among blacks and to 67 percent among white Appalachians. Similarly, one third of non-Appalachian whites are employed in professional, technical, or managerial occupations, but only 19 percent of blacks and only 8 percent of white Appalachians hold such positions. Whereas 22 percent of the non-Appalachian whites report annual family incomes of $40,000 or more, only 16 percent of blacks and 7 percent of white Appalachians have incomes at this level. Although the Appalachians' lower socioeconomic status is attributable in part to the higher percentage of females in this group, it is evident that Appalachians living in the city have a low socioeconomic status overall. As a group, they are closer to blacks in these characteristics than to non-Appalachian whites (Obermiller and Oldendick 1987).

Some Appalachians in greater Cincinnati are black. Black Appalachians have somewhat less education but earn slightly more income and enjoy higher occupational status than do other blacks in Cincinnati. Yet these differences become inconsequential when compared with the much larger differences between blacks and whites in the city. Overall the socioeconomic resemblance of black Appalachians to other blacks is much stronger than the similarities between white Appalachians and other whites. Black Appalachians have assimilated into the urban black community to a degree that white Appalachians have not achieved with reference to the larger white community in Cincinnati (Philliber and Obermiller 1982).

Like black Appalachians, Appalachian women form a minority within a minority in urban areas. Although nearly four fifths of urban Appalachian women work full-time, they are less educated, hold lower-status jobs, and live in households earning less average annual income than do their male counterparts. The subordinate status of Appalachians in greater Cincinnati seems to intensify the stratification between Appalachian men and women (Community Chest and Council of the Cincinnati Area 1983).

A TALE OF TWO CITIES: PITTSBURGH

The steady decline of the steel industry over the past 60 years has directly affected Pittsburgh's demographic profile. The story has been one of outmigration rather than inmigration; the Steel City has lost 80,000 industrial jobs and more than 90,000 residents in the last two decades. Between 1980 and 1989 the Pittsburgh metropolitan area experienced the largest population decrease recorded for any U.S. metropolis. The city's demographic losses are the highest in the nation, whether considered in terms of net population loss (134,200) or as a percentage of total population (5.7%) (Bangs and Singh 1988).

According to research on Appalachian migration to Pittsburgh based on 1960 and 1970 census data, Pittsburgh was not a popular destination for migrants from southern Appalachia (McCoy and Brown 1981). In 1960, Pittsburgh was ranked twenty-seventh out of the 30 top-ranked metropolitan destinations for Appalachian migration; by 1970, it had dropped to twenty-ninth and was ranked a distant last among the seven metropolitan receiving areas located in the Appalachian region.

Surprisingly, the 1980 figures on Appalachian mobility reveal Pittsburgh as the first of the 30 top-ranked metropolitan receiving areas (Obermiller and Oldendick 1987). Even so, we must keep several factors in mind when interpreting these data. First, in *net* Appalachian migration (the number of people entering Pittsburgh from elsewhere in Appalachia minus the number of people leaving Pittsburgh for some other destination in Appalachia), Pittsburgh actually lost 1,789 migrants in 1980. Second, the 1960 and 1970 data consider only migrants from southern Appalachia; they disregard those from Appalachian counties in New York, Ohio, and Pennsylvania. Those statistics excluded the ring of Appalachian counties surrounding Allegheny County, whereas these counties were included in the migration data for 1980. Indeed, a close examination of the more recent data shows that the Appalachian counties of southwestern Pennsylvania are the primary sources of Appalachian migration to Pittsburgh; they contributed nearly one third of all migrants to Pittsburgh in 1980. The balance of the Appalachian migrants came principally from the Appalachian counties of western Pennsylvania, southwestern New York, and southeastern Ohio; migrants from West Virginia are a fairly small part of this migration stream.

Pittsburgh, like Cincinnati, is a city of neighborhoods. Natives and visitors alike are keenly aware of this reality; one gives and receives directions that begin with statements like "That's in Oakland" or "Take the Liberty Bridge over to Mt. Washington." In both cities natural neighborhood boundaries such as rivers, hills, and ravines are supplemented by parks, boulevards, and railway tracks.

Long-established ethnic group settlement patterns give Pittsburgh residents a clear idea of who lives where (Bodnar, Simon, and Weber 1982). Polish Hill, of course, is Polish. Bloomfield is heavily Italian. Much of the city's black population lives in the Hill district northeast of downtown. Squirrel Hill is heavily Jewish. Oakland, near the city's major universities and hospitals, is diverse and cosmopolitan. Large-

scale outmigration of blue-collar families since 1970 has weakened but
has not destroyed these ethnic enclaves. Gentrification has occurred in
some areas, but these demographic changes will not soon alter basic
neighborhood characteristics based on ethnicity and social class.

The area has suffered severely from loss of population and of blue-
collar jobs, but Pittsburgh's ethnic neighborhoods remain intact,
primarily through the resilience of their residents. In the past, three
generations of working-class families in ethnic neighborhoods usually
occupied three separate houses in their community. These families now
are doubling and tripling up in one house. As one informant told the
authors, "Grandma moved in, and the kids are staying or moving back
in." Family income lost in the former industrial economy is replaced
partially through informal exchanges and casual labor, the "off the
books" transactions such as flea market sales, odd jobs, repair work, and
babysitting. One informant reported, "The jobs are not here to support
the yuppies the city seeks. The ethnic neighborhoods are safe."

Home ownership is another factor in the relative stability of
Pittsburgh's neighborhoods. Nationally, the home ownership rate is 63.8
percent; in Pittsburgh, it is 74.4 percent. Moreover, housing in this area is
less expensive than in other U.S. cities. Only 4 of the 150 largest cities in
the country have average housing costs lower than Pittsburgh's.

The existence of ethnic neighborhoods is not enough in itself to
explain why West Virginians and other Appalachians have not
established their own neighborhoods in Pittsburgh. Ethnic succession in
urban neighborhoods is a fact of life in most major metropolitan areas; in
1940, for example, several inner-city neighborhoods in Cincinnati were
primarily German Catholic or Jewish; by 1970, these neighborhoods
were predominantly Appalachian or black. Yet this process, which took
place in Cincinnati and other midwestern cities, apparently did not occur
in Pittsburgh, although the circumstances in Pittsburgh were as
conducive to succession as in other cities.

In Cincinnati, Appalachians are the largest resident group in at least
10 neighborhoods. They are organized politically and culturally,
operating several community centers and celebrating their culture with
local and regional festivals. Cincinnati is the location of the Frank Foster
Library on Appalachian Migrants as well as the home of the Urban
Appalachian Council, the Appalachian People's Service Organization,
and the Appalachian Community Development Association. Appalachian
churches can be found across the city and (more frequently in recent
years) in the suburbs. Urban Appalachians have gained recognition by
city government, the school board, and community social agencies as
Cincinnati's second largest minority group after blacks.

Blue-collar Appalachians are a major part of the work force in local factories; their white-collar counterparts work in hospitals, schools, and social service agencies across the metropolitan area. Urban health care delivery systems are learning to adapt to the special needs of Appalachian migrants, such as screening and treatment for pneumoconiosis. As early as the 1970s the superintendent of the Cincinnati Public Schools stated that serving the educational needs of Appalachian students was one of the most serious challenges facing the school system.

Because one of every four residents has Appalachian roots, Cincinnati has long been a focal point for academic research on patterns of internal migration, urban social problems, and ethnic group formation. The research has resulted in numerous journal articles, at least four scholarly books, several novels, and the organization of Appalachian studies courses at local colleges and universities.

No such expressions of an Appalachian presence can be found in Pittsburgh. On our visits the residents easily gave us directions to other ethnic neighborhoods in the city, but no one could direct us to an Appalachian neighborhood, to a "hillbilly" bar or restaurant, or to a preacher with an Appalachian congregation.

We visited poor white neighborhoods in and around the city. The central institutions located in these neighborhoods—grocery stores, bars, and churches—stocked no Appalachian food on their shelves, played no bluegrass music on their jukeboxes, and included no traditional mountain hymns in their services. We checked for West Virginia plates on cars and trucks in driveways and on the streets. We looked for Churches of Christ and Holiness churches. We listened for regional accents on the streets and asked people whether they knew of anybody from West Virginia living in the area. All to no avail. All of the people we spoke with were technically "Appalachian" in the sense that they lived in the federally defined region. Some no doubt are rural-to-urban migrants, but we found no evidence of large concentrations of people who had migrated from the mountains of West Virginia or who could be considered culturally Appalachian.

Even in the steel towns along the Monongahela and the Ohio rivers, we received the impression from our interviews that West Virginian migrants were relatively invisible. They settled in, socialized among themselves, and got along peaceably enough with their Croatian and Polish neighbors. They did not, however, take over large sections of the towns or build any permanent edifices equivalent to the domed and spired churches of the European immigrants. Perhaps a typical pattern was that the first-generation migrants moved back to West Virginia to retire, and their children, second-generation migrants, moved on to other midwestern cities as the decline in the steel industry grew more severe.

HYPOTHESES

There are many possible explanations for the different outcomes of Appalachian migration to Pittsburgh and to Cincinnati. The first we call the spatial argument: Pittsburgh offered no physical, social, or economic space to the newcomers. Tight-knit ethnic neighborhoods of blacks, Croatians, Poles, Italians, and other groups prevented the relatively late-arriving Appalachians from establishing a toehold in the city. These ethnically homogeneous communities had been maintained over time because individual houses often were inherited by family members or sold to neighbors. The same consistency typified the blue-collar job market in Pittsburgh; working-class ethnics controlled the unions and the lower-management positions, ensuring that new hires would come from their own networks of kin, neighbors, and friends. The abiding solidarity of early migrants to Pittsburgh may have acted to exclude Appalachian newcomers from communities, housing, and jobs.

Another, similar explanation is based on the nature of ethnic group behavior. Patterns of ethnic clustering by occupation and industry have been well documented. Groups not only are excluded from occupational opportunities but also self-segregate in the labor force through ethnically specific job search patterns and employment preferences. According to this view, Appalachian workers in the Midwest gravitated toward the automobile industry rather than the steel industry, for whatever reason. This tendency would account for the presence of large numbers of Appalachians living in Cleveland, Detroit, Chicago, and Cincinnati as well as for their absence in Pittsburgh. (We know of only one exception to this pattern—at Armco Steel in Middletown, Ohio—but most of Armco's output is consumed by the automobile industry.) This theory also is supported by the recruitment practices of industries; having found a reliable and satisfactory source of labor, they tend to tap it again and again.

A third possible explanation for the absence of Appalachian neighborhoods in Pittsburgh is a variation of the ethnic argument. That is, the migrants to Pittsburgh from the Appalachian region are themselves of immigrant stock and have blended quietly into the various ethnic communities in the city. The urban Appalachians in Pittsburgh may have been miners of Italian and Polish descent from the Appalachian coalfields of southwestern Pennsylvania. These ethnic miners may have moved to Pittsburgh to become steelworkers. Evidence supporting this ethnic argument comes from the recent migration data for Allegheny County cited above.

From a different viewpoint, we can hypothesize that Cincinnati and Pittsburgh experienced two different kinds of migration streams from Appalachia. Unlike the fairly direct moves from the region to midwestern cities such as Chicago, Detroit, and Cincinnati, the flow to Pittsburgh may have been interrupted by diffusion. In short, migrants coming up the Monongahela Valley or across the upper Ohio River Valley may have encountered intervening opportunities in the mill towns south and west of Pittsburgh. The opportunity to avoid the big city, combined with job opportunities closer to "home" in West Virginia and southeastern Ohio, may have siphoned off many potential migrants to Pittsburgh. In a variation of this idea, the migrants may have stopped short of Pittsburgh and may have taken up residence in the ring of counties surrounding the city. By commuting, these migrants could participate in the city's labor force while retaining some semblance of rural life. This line of thinking gains credence from the presence of a large white Protestant underclass in towns such as Beaver Falls, Aliquippa, and Washington. These people, living in Appalachia as defined by the federal government, display some Appalachian cultural characteristics and in fact may have been among the earliest Appalachian migrants to the area.

Another set of explanations comes from an understanding of the respective economic and social structures of the two cities. The long-term decline of the steel industry and the concomitant downward trend in the Pittsburgh area economy began in the 1930s and was reversed only briefly by World War II. The area may never have attracted migrant workers as strongly as industrial cities not dependent on steel, such as Cincinnati, Baltimore, and Columbus.

Social mobility also was limited in Pittsburgh by an enduring working class. In Cincinnati, by contrast, working-class Germans moved into the middle and upper classes, providing blue-collar Appalachian migrants with an opportunity to move into the neighborhoods, housing, and jobs that the Germans left behind. Thousands of Cincinnati Germans, for example, joined the postwar movement to the suburbs. One neighborhood, Lower Price Hill, was predominantly German in 1940; by 1960, it was almost entirely white Appalachian. The stagnant economy of Pittsburgh, on the other hand, inhibited mobility in the social and economic structures of the city.

Does this situation mean that Pittsburgh's current efforts to move from blue-collar to white-collar industries will create new social and occupational opportunities for Appalachian migrants? We think not. Jobs in the primary and secondary industrial sectors are vanishing, even as jobs in the tertiary sector are being created. Ethnic succession in Pittsburgh's labor force and neighborhoods is less likely to occur than the social immobility caused by the decline in blue-collar work.

Which of these hypotheses accounts most accurately for the absence of Appalachians in Pittsburgh? Probably all of them, in some combination. As observers from Cincinnati, we have raised the question and have brought it to this point. Now it is time for students of Pittsburgh's history to take up the task, to examine the historical evidence for each of the hypotheses we have offered, and to determine their relative importance.

3

The Sense of Place and Cultural Identity among Urban Appalachians: A Study in Postdeath Migration

Phillip J. Obermiller and Ray Rappold

Cultural patterns historically have determined the disposition of human remains. Early Christians placed their dead in catacombs in anticipation of Jesus's imminent return and the Final Judgment. In the seventh century, Christians began the custom of interments in hallowed grounds: churchyards for peasants and cathedral crypts for princes and popes. The glorification of nature in the Renaissance gave rise to the parklike rural cemetery familiar in modern times, and the environmental concerns of the late twentieth century have made cremation a popular alternative to traditional burial (Phipps 1989; Smith 1988).

In Appalachia, cultural preferences and environmental constraints have affected the disposition of the dead. The family graveyard high on a mountainside is still a familiar sight across the region (Wigginton 1973). Even the larger cemeteries in churchyards or near main roads in Appalachia show signs of frequent visitation: carefully tended plots and displays of flowers, wreaths, and flags. These cemeteries can be viewed as symbols of the Appalachian people's relationship to the land, an important part of the "sense of place" discussed in the recent literature (Center for Appalachian Studies and Services 1989; Whitson 1988). This sense of place, however, has been threatened by the mass migrations from the Appalachian region that have occurred over the past 50 years (Obermiller and Oldendick 1987).

It is possible to investigate migrants' attachment to their places of origin in a variety of ways. Shuttle migration, frequent visits or vacations "down home," monetary remittances, subscriptions to hometown newspapers, absentee voting, and patterns of letter writing and long-distance calling are all valid indicators of migrants' residual allegiance to specific places.

How strong is the attachment to a homeplace among urban Appalachians? To answer this question, we selected the place of interment as a surrogate for sense of place in Appalachia and analyzed patterns of Appalachian postdeath migration. In addition, through an examination of funeral practices, we investigated the strength of Appalachian customs and culture among urban Appalachians who do not return family members to the region for burial.

DATA AND ANALYSIS

Our data on burial come from three sources: content analysis of obituaries published recently in a large-circulation West Virginia newspaper, analysis of a sample of death certificates provided by a funeral livery service that links southwestern Ohio with eastern Kentucky, and interviews with key informants such as the operators of funeral homes serving large Appalachian migrant communities in Ohio.

Obituaries

No state or county in the nation keeps records on the inflow of human remains for burial (Rowles and Comeaux 1987). This information can be found, however, in the obituary notices of Appalachian newspapers such as the *Charleston Gazette*, a West Virginia newspaper with a relatively large circulation (54,804). The paper's daily obituary column provides local, statewide, and out-of-state coverage, as well as information on bodies being returned to West Virginia for burial.

In the six-month period between August 1989 and January 1990, 4,478 obituaries were published in the *Gazette*; of these, 471 (10.5%) documented the demise of native West Virginians who were living in other states at the time of their deaths. More than two thirds of these deaths occurred in five states: Ohio accounted for 25.5 percent of the out-of-state deaths; Florida, for 21.2 percent; Virginia, for 10.6 percent; and Texas and Maryland, for 5 percent each. In 267 (56.7%) of the obituaries documenting out-of-state deaths, it was stated that a body was being returned to West Virginia for burial.

According to these figures, well over half of the West Virginians who die outside the state are returned to the mountains for burial. This proportion, however, is exaggerated by the fact that the *Gazette* publishes only the out-of-state obituaries that are provided to it. Out-of-state families returning kin for interment make arrangements through West Virginia funeral directors, who notify the local papers. Many out-of-state families who do not return relatives for burial have little or no incentive to notify the newspapers in the region; they also lack access to the routine notification mechanisms used by funeral directors. In short, the West Virginia obituaries reflect accurately the number of returns but most likely understate the number of former residents who die and are buried outside the state. The true proportion of returns is probably much smaller than the one-in-two ratio suggested by the obituaries.

In addition, there may be nothing particularly "Appalachian" about the large number of returns from Florida to West Virginia documented by the obituaries. Florida and Arizona are recognized as desirable relocation sites for retirees from across the country; therefore, both Appalachian and non-Appalachian migrants who die in either of these states are quite likely to be returned to their state of origin for burial (Rowles and Comeaux 1986, 1987).

Death Certificates

The transportation of bodies over long distances became practical earlier in this century with the advent of modern embalming techniques and express trains (Shneidman 1976). The military developed international air delivery systems for war casualties to such an extent that there are no American military cemeteries in Korea or in Vietnam (Rowles and Comeaux 1987). Jessica Mitford (1963) estimated that 10 percent of all funerals in the United States involve this type of long-distance "removal." Funeral directors generally cannot spare the personnel, equipment, or time needed for the long-distance delivery of bodies. Usually, they turn to commercial livery firms that specialize in carrying human remains. One such firm is the C&C Mortuary Service, located in Covington, Kentucky. Operated by a father-and-son team who migrated to the area from the mountains of eastern Kentucky, C&C provides transport services for many of the funeral homes in greater Cincinnati. Analysis of the records (copies of death certificates) kept by C&C over the five-year period 1985 through 1989 shows that 332 (31%) of the 1,077 cases handled by the firm were removals from the greater Cincinnati area to the Appalachian region. As might be expected, eastern Kentucky accounted for 88 percent of the returns to Appalachian counties; West Virginia, Virginia, and Pennsylvania together accounted for another 10 percent; Tennessee, Ohio, and New York received the balance (Catchen 1989).

Analysis of the data taken from the death certificates shows that nearly one third of the out-of-state burials from greater Cincinnati take place in the Appalachian region. Most interments from this area occur in eastern Kentucky; many of these burials are in family graveyards rather than in public or nonprofit private cemeteries. Males and females are equally likely to be returned to the region for burial.

Information obtained from this sample of death certificates, however, does not tell us what proportion of all Appalachians who die are returned to the mountains for burial. Because the death certificates usually indicate only the decedent's state of birth, it is nearly impossible to produce a reliable figure on mortality rates among urban Appalachians. As a result, we lack the denominator necessary to compute the actual proportion of returns among Appalachians. Hence, the figure (31%) obtained from the death certificates provides no reliable basis for determining sense of place among urban Appalachians when interment is used as the variable.

Interviews

We chose two cities in Butler County, Ohio, as sites for interviews because of their size and their large Appalachian populations. Middletown has a population of 43,719, and Hamilton has a population of 63,189; unofficial estimates place the Appalachian migrant population in each city at about 60 percent.

To select informants for interviews in each city, we used the reputational method. First we consulted the National Directory of Morticians (1989) for a list of all funeral homes in the two cities and phoned each one, explaining our research interest. Then we selected the funeral director in each city whom colleagues named consistently as serving a large number of Appalachian families.

William Riggs is a third-generation funeral director and a first-generation Appalachian migrant from West Virginia. The Riggs Funeral Home, the oldest in Middletown, oversees approximately 60 burials a year. Riggs estimates that about 75 percent of his trade comes from families with roots in eastern Kentucky; fewer than 10 percent of his Appalachian cases, however, are returned to the region for interment. Riggs points out that as many as half of the latter are "round trippers," elderly people in failing health brought from the mountains to Middletown for care by their families before their demise. He notes that long-term residents who are returned to the mountains for burial tend to belong to an earlier generation of migrants; with very few exceptions, second- and third-generation urban Appalachians who die in Middletown are buried locally (Riggs 1990).

George Brown is a second-generation funeral director with no roots in Appalachia. His firm, however, the Brown-Dawson Funeral Home in Hamilton, counts a "nearly 100 percent" Appalachian clientele among the 300 funerals it conducts in an average year. Like Riggs, Brown also estimates a 10 percent return rate, primarily to eastern Kentucky. He also points out that many of the returns involve elderly, short-term residents of Hamilton. It is his perception that the rate of returns is diminishing over time and is limited to an older generation of migrants (G. Brown 1990).

Dr. Dan Flory, president of the Cincinnati College of Mortuary Science at Xavier University, is a former partner in his father-in-law's Middletown firm, the Breitenbach McCoy-Leffler Funeral Home. Flory was mentioned frequently by the funeral directors we contacted as having both a local and a national perspective on his profession. His independent estimate of the removals from greater Cincinnati to eastern Kentucky (10%) was quite consistent with the other responses we received (Flory 1990).

The funeral directors we interviewed provided an important insight: in most cases, returning a body to the Appalachian region is less expensive than local interment. The average cost of returning a body from Cincinnati to a family-owned plot in eastern Kentucky (including burial) is about $300. In the Middletown area, similar costs for burial in a prepurchased grave average about $715 (Riggs 1990). Economic factors therefore are not a deterrent to returns among low-income families.

The estimates we obtained from interviews with the key informants appear to provide the most dependable assessment of Appalachians' return to their home region after death. The funeral directors estimated consistently and independently that 1 Appalachian migrant in 10 is returned to the region for burial. They also placed this figure in context by stating that perhaps half of these persons were not true migrants but were involved in a process that has been described in the literature as relocation due to deteriorating health (Rowles 1983) or "mobility for chronic assistance" (Meyer and Cromley 1989). Therefore, this 10 percent estimate should be reduced by half because the frail elderly persons who may have lived all but the last few months of their lives in Appalachia never had the opportunity to redefine "home" in the same way as long-term migrants. According to the adjusted estimates, then, only about 5 percent of the burials conducted by funeral directors serving distinctly Appalachian clienteles involve true attachment to place. Moreover, these typically are the funerals of persons in the oldest age cohort in the migrant community; as a consequence, the overall number of returns to the region is declining over time.

Funeral Customs

Migrants may not be returned to the region for burial in meaningful numbers; yet wherever the burial takes place, Appalachians' consistent adherence to particular funeral customs makes them easily identifiable as a distinctive cultural group. To make this point, we return to the information provided by the funeral directors.

The first piece of evidence is the most obvious: like Jews, blacks, Italians, and members of other ethnic minorities, Appalachian families take their trade to specific funeral homes. They do so because these firms are familiar with the funeral customs of the people they serve and are willing to meet their special requirements. For instance, many Appalachian blue-collar workers in Hamilton have union contracts that allow up to three days' paid leave of absence for the death of a family member. The funeral home serving Appalachians in Hamilton routinely distributes specially printed cards that provide employers with the information required to activate the leave of absence (G. Brown 1990).

Our interview informants were aware of practices that distinguish Appalachian funeral services from others. Appalachians prefer long visiting hours, beginning at the time of death, when the undertaker may be delayed in removing the body until all family members have gathered to pay their respects. Another characteristic is an almost complete avoidance of practices that are increasingly commonplace in the general population, such as autopsies to ascertain cause of death, harvesting usable organs from the body, donating the body for medical research, and cremation.

Another important aspect of Appalachian funeral services is the role of religion. One preacher and sometimes two will conduct a funeral service lasting up to three hours. The funeral directors observe that the preachers, beyond their spiritual dimension, are highly skilled in assisting bereaved families to face and release their grief (Hager 1989). One informant noted that Appalachians, with the help of their clergy, are particularly good at working through the grief process (Flory 1990).

Floral tributes are regarded as an important part of an urban Appalachian funeral; alternatives such as making donations to a favorite charity in lieu of sending flowers are usually not offered. Typical floral arrangements at an urban Appalachian funeral may include a wheel with one spoke missing or a telephone with the receiver off the hook and the words "Jesus Has Called." Informants also noted customs such as placing family photographs or other meaningful items in the coffin and bringing the deceased person's favorite chair to the funeral home and allowing it to stand symbolically empty (G. Brown 1990).

The funeral is an important social occasion for urban Appalachian families. As news of the death spreads, the funeral director is inundated with calls not only about the hours of visitation but also about who is expected to attend from out of town. Calling hours at the funeral home provide an opportunity for friends and acquaintances of the family, as well as family members themselves, to visit and catch up on each other's lives. "Marryin's and buryin's" in the urban Appalachian community generally involve large meals as well. After the services are completed, guests are invited to a meal at home or at a local church, where the visiting continues unabated (G. Brown 1990).

DISCUSSION AND CONCLUSION

The rate of removals to the Appalachian region is small and appears to be declining. Our findings on postdeath migration reveal that most urban Appalachians have transferred their sense of "home" from the mountains to the cities in which they now reside. Even so, they maintain funeral customs that distinguish them clearly from other urban cultural groups.

Initially, we wished to learn whether migrants from Appalachia to urban areas outside the region have assimilated so completely into the urban milieu that they lose their identification with their home region. In attempting to answer this question, we discovered the distinction between being "geographically Appalachian" and being "socially Appalachian." According to our evidence, it seems possible to be Appalachian without thinking of the region as home. Although many Appalachian migrants think fondly or nostalgically about their place of origin, they have transferred their sense of place to their new neighborhoods and communities (Kemme, 1990). Urban Appalachians are now "at home" in neighborhood social networks of their coworkers, friends, neighbors, children, and grandchildren. These people are no longer Appalachian in a geographical sense, but they maintain cultural practices that make them unmistakably Appalachian in a social sense.

It appears from this analysis that Appalachian postdeath migration is a relatively minor phenomenon, restricted to a particular age cohort that is shrinking. Although we use postdeath migration to indicate sense of place, most Appalachian migrants and their families have found a new homeplace, and it is not in Appalachia. Nonetheless, they remain very much Appalachian.

4

Appalachian Women: Between Two Cultures

H. Virginia McCoy, Diana Gullett Trevino, and Clyde B. McCoy

Ethnic, minority, and cultural groups are generally perceived by others as homogeneous. It is true that groups have characteristics that bind them together and cause them to be recognized as groups. Within the group, however, members have distinctive characteristics that display their heterogeneity. Appalachians are such a group.

Both women's roles and identification with a cultural group have consequences for opportunities in mainstream society. Social characteristics such as gender, ethnicity, and race tend to be associated with differences in access to economic rewards and to those available in education, in personal power, and in political power.

This chapter explores Appalachian migrant women's roles in the Appalachian community, using a framework developed by Davidson and Gordon (1979). Although researchers differ as to whether Appalachians are an ethnic group (Branscome 1976; Obermiller 1977; Walls 1976), they exhibit sufficient differences from other groups (other migrants, natives, blacks) to justify study as an ethnic group (Philliber 1981b). Davidson and Gordon's framework provides a useful theoretical model for analyzing the situation of Appalachian migrant women. It addresses the development of gender roles as they are influenced by three social factors:

1. The group's position in the stratification system, which will determine their access to the rewards and opportunities available in the social system.
2. The cultural heritage of the group, which will determine those values, beliefs, and behaviors (i.e., gender roles) that are acceptable within the group, as well as coping mechanisms

needed to adjust to the new environment. Traditional behaviors and beliefs may have to be modified to fulfill roles and behaviors that are acceptable in the new setting. The existence of an ethnic community provides a mechanism for making these adjustments. Group members' participation in the ethnic community will provide the support system necessary to make these adjustments in order to attain the rewards and opportunities available to the larger society.

3. The degree to which group members identify with their ethnic group, which will determine "their ideal versions of a role as well as their extent of participation in an ethnic environment supportive of any given role" (Davidson and Gordon 1979, p. 126).

SOCIAL INFLUENCES ON APPALACHIAN WOMEN'S GENDER ROLES

Appalachians' Position in the Stratification System

Empirical studies have shown that Appalachian migrants occupy a low status in the stratification hierarchy in urban areas. Their occupational status is lower than that of other groups, either other migrants or natives. They are concentrated in unskilled or semiskilled jobs; and few hold professional or managerial positions (Philliber 1981a, 1981b; Photiadis 1981; Schwarzweller 1981; Schwarzweller, Brown, and Mangalam 1971).

In addition, Appalachians receive the lowest income increases attained for concomitant increases in occupational status (Philliber 1981b). The literature on Appalachian employment status shows that, in general, Appalachians are able to find jobs and are willing to take lower-status jobs (Philliber 1981b; Photiadis 1981; Schwarzweller, Brown, and Mangalam 1971). Most studies of migration find that fewer Appalachian women than their urban counterparts work outside the home (Philliber 1981b; Powles 1978); a greater number, however, are employed than among Appalachians who remain in the mountains (Schwarzweller, Brown, and Mangalam 1971). About one third of women in the Beech Creek study worked outside the home in teaching and clerical positions; most, however, held semiskilled or unskilled jobs (Schwarzweller, Brown, and Mangalam 1971, p. 143). Only one study of recent Appalachian migrant females suggested that they are not disadvantaged in the economic domain (Watkins and Trevino 1982).

Political power is another measure of a group's position in the stratification system. Appalachians as a group have not been viewed as a political force in cities; they do not have many identifiable representatives in government, nor do they vote as a bloc. In fact, fewer Appalachians than other white migrants, white natives, or blacks are registered to vote in Hamilton County, Ohio (Cincinnati), and they vote less frequently than the other groups (Philliber 1981b).

Appalachians' position in the stratification system thus places them at a disadvantage in obtaining the rewards and opportunities available to the majority society. In this respect, Appalachian women are subject to the same constraints as Appalachian men. Their social position affects other group members as well as the next generation. Their status as women within the culture, however, places an additional restriction on their opportunities, as will become evident in the next section.

The Appalachian Community

The second factor that affects gender roles in ethnic groups is the existence of an ethnic community that assists in providing the support mechanisms for coping with the new environment. The majority of Appalachians in Cincinnati originally settled in low-income, inner-city Appalachian neighborhoods (Fowler 1981), but later studies suggest that many Appalachians also live in the suburbs (Philliber 1981b). The existence of an Appalachian community is evidenced by its size and by the recognition it receives from observers, as well as by the establishment of Appalachian neighborhoods. The kinship network is the support mechanism used by recent Appalachian migrants in adjusting to the urban environment. Schwarzweller, Brown, and Mangalam (1971) recognize that family members in the new community and in the home neighborhood provide support to migrants in the form of information about jobs, doctors, where to shop, and acceptable behavior.

Although the maintenance of ideal cultural norms may depend on the existence of a sizable ethnic community, the members must learn new roles that are more compatible with the new setting. Appalachians brought to the cities their traditional beliefs and values. Life in the isolation of the Appalachian hills produced the kinds of beliefs and values that were suitable to survival in the wilderness.

In the traditional patriarchal structure of Appalachian families, the husband was the leader and made the economic, social, and familial decisions (Schwarzweller, Brown, and Mangalam 1971). Mountain women were responsible for child-rearing, health care, carrying water from the spring, making and mending clothes, processing food, tending the garden, preparing meals, and all other domestic chores (Campbell 1921). Young girls were trained to follow in their mothers' footsteps. It was a hard, demanding life: "At twenty the mountain woman is old in all that makes a woman old—toil, sorrow, childbearing, loneliness and pitiful want" (Miles 1905).

Although the patriarchal culture in Appalachia placed women in a secondary status, elderly women had a special position. They carried on the family's health care traditions; many were "granny women" who knew of herbs and teas to cure almost any ailment. They received respect for their wisdom and knowledge. With increasing age, women attained positions of authority and recognition; their advice was freely given and accepted, even by their husbands: "She...gained a freedom and a place of irresponsible authority in the home hardly rivaled by the men of the family....In old age she [attained] the dignity of labor achieved" (Campbell 1921, p. 140).

Contemporary Appalachian women follow patterns similar to those of their sisters in earlier times. Pat Beaver describes the social system of rural eastern Tennessee, in which cooperation between men and women is a necessary ingredient yet in which duties are carried out according to gender:

The female domestic sphere includes primary responsibility for the care and socialization of children, and for household and garden maintenance; the male extra-domestic sphere includes all things not related to child care and household and garden maintenance. However, these role structures are flexible in the sense that pragmatism, a dominant cultural theme in a historically and economically tenuous environment, may require constant adjustment. (Beaver 1979, p. 66)

There is some indication, as Beaver suggests, that although current gender roles still are limited by women's subordinate status with respect to males, these roles are undergoing changes similar to those in the mainstream society. According to McKenry, Reed, and Knipers (1979, p. 75), a majority (74%) of their eastern Tennessee respondents believe that household duties should be shared equally; they do not put this belief into practice, however. The status of Appalachian women in society depends on their power. Beaver (1979) recognized that although Appalachian women possess no formal access to power, they have some informal sources: (1) their ability to get things done, (2) their manipulation of men, and (3) their increasing influence as they age. Additional sources of power within the authority structure of Appalachian families may offer other avenues to women as well. A Tennessee study (McKenry

1979) found that wives appear to be making more family household decisions than generally believed:

Husbands were perceived in the traditional role of the main source of authority, making the most important decisions. However, by examining husband and wife disagreements, it appears that the husband does not exercise much more power than the wife in getting his way. (McKenry 1979, p. 77)

Also, in arguments with children, husbands fared less well than did wives or children.

Although the roles and status of Appalachian women in the mountains apparently are changing, the process of migration places the women in circumstances that necessitate changes in their roles upon arrival in the city. Social scientists have neglected the roles, conflicts, and circumstances of the women who took part in the "great migration" from Appalachia in the 1940s, 1950s, and 1960s. Most of these women came with their husbands or parents or joined other relatives who came to industrial cities in search of jobs and a better life. Appalachian women brought with them the cultural heritage of their sisters who stayed behind; migration, however, forced changes in the culture.

Harriet Arnow's *The Dollmaker* (1954) provides a vivid, although fictional, account of the stress and hardships that Gertie Nevel experienced in leaving her beloved land and adjusting to the urban life of Detroit.

It is a moving and positive as well as sensitive portrayal of a woman who moved to the confusing city world....Gertie and her family face prejudice, hassles for money, insensitive institutions and the penalties for trying to maintain a unique identity. (Trevino 1978, p. 111)

The limited social science literature indicates that the social adjustment process required of Appalachian migrant women produces greater change in them than in the men. Appalachian culture requires that women fulfill the traditional roles of homemaker and mother, but the urban setting demands some transformation in decision making, in employment, and in marital relationships.

An exploratory study of Appalachian migrants conducted during the 1950s briefly mentions the women's roles in the family. Giffin (1954) suggests that the time required to perform the traditional tasks of growing and processing food, preparing meals, and caring for the home decreased for Appalachian migrant women. The restricted space and the expanded technology of the urban setting reduced the importance of many of these tasks. Women then adjusted their efforts to focus on caring for their children.

Decision making among Appalachian migrants is primarily the husband's responsibility. The 1961 Beech Creek study found that both men and women perceive the husband as the chief decision maker in family affairs. The husband's realm includes not only major decisions, such as the decision to migrate, but also daily activities (Schwarzweller, Brown, and Mangalam 1971). Powles (1978) suggests that changes in roles produced conflicts between husbands and wives. Urban wives traditionally were responsible for relating to the community in such activities as shopping, attending PTA meetings, and church activities. The Appalachian patriarchal family structure, however, demanded that the husband make decisions on such matters. "This disruption in the traditional balance of power included practical consequences. For example, the Appalachian workingman will be highly suspicious at first of any community agency which deals with his wife 'behind his back' while he is at work" (Powles 1978, p. 181).

In regard to men's authoritative role, Appalachian migrants' attitudes apparently have changed little since the 1950s and 1960s. A 1979 survey of northern Kentucky residents found that 82 percent of Appalachian migrants, 54 percent of second-generation Appalachians, 47 percent of other migrants, 25 percent of second-generation other migrants, and 41 percent of long-term residents believe that women should not have authority over men, even in areas where the women are better qualified (Traina 1980).

Among second-generation Appalachians, however, belief in the subordinate role of women appears to be changing. Traditional roles that were acceptable in the mountains apparently have been found less helpful in the urban environment. The migrants have had to learn new behaviors to facilitate adjustment and to gain access to the opportunities available in the new setting.

Attitudes about women's roles in work have received some attention in the literature. Eighty-three percent of Appalachians in northern Kentucky believe that women should not work to support the family, compared with 50 percent of other migrants and 42 percent of long-term residents (Traina 1980). These attitudes reflect cultural beliefs and behaviors in the Appalachian family. The belief that women should remain in the home and should not participate in the paid work force endures among Appalachian migrants; however, situations have forced them to alter their behavior to fit the new setting.

Identification as Appalachians

Davidson and Gordon's third social influence on gender roles in ethnic groups concerns the identification of group members with their cultural heritage. The extent to which Appalachians identify and participate with other Appalachians should support traditional or nontraditional roles. T. Miller (1978) found that more than one third of Appalachians in a survey in Norwood, Ohio, identified themselves as Appalachians. She argues that this proportion is sizable in view of the stage of development of Appalachian urban identity. Davidson's model suggests that the greater the self-identification with the ethnic group, the greater the likelihood that roles acceptable in the culture will be supported and continued. The level of self-identification among Appalachians suggests that there should be opportunity for changes in traditional roles. Yet we also must consider other definitions and recognition of the group. An individual's identification with an ethnic group "is subject to the definitions and constraints imposed externally by others" (Davidson and Gordon 1979, p. 126). In addition, Horowitz (1975) contends that there may be a lag time in which self-identification and identification of others are placed on the group. T. Miller (1978) argues that this is the situation with Appalachians: more than 40 percent of non-Appalachians in her study identified Appalachians as an ethnic group. The lag time in identification of the group, coupled with negative stereotypes associated with Appalachians, probably inhibits their self-identification with the group.

Appalachian women have been unduly stereotyped for many years. The Daisy Mae, Mammy Yokum, and (more recently) Dolly Parton images invoked by the words *hillbilly woman* have forced Appalachian women either to defend or to conceal their heritage. Kahn (1973) and Lord and Patton-Crowder (1979) describe the actions and thoughts of women who exemplify the heterogeneity of Appalachia: Granny Hager's struggle to obtain black lung benefits, and her subsequent advocacy of those rights for others; a college professor's ambitions to become a college president; the socialization of an Appalachian feminist; and the Wilson and Chandler women's efforts to adjust to the confinements and abuses of city life. We must come to understand both the commonalities and the differences among Appalachian women: "We must define ourselves and not accept hand-me-down stereotypes" (Trevino 1978, p. 111).

Schwarzweller, Brown, and Mangalam (1971) suggest that both the women who worked outside the home and the full-time homemakers who lived outside "hillbilly neighborhoods" had more contacts with native Ohioans than did males, and this association hastened the women's assimilation into urban life. Men tended to work in factories with many other Appalachians, so their cultural ties to the mountains remained stronger.

While the process of social absorption into the urban community may be more rapid for women as compared with men, they may feel more alienated from the mountain way of life. In that sense, they encounter greater, or at least different, adjustment problems from those encountered by men. (Schwarzweller, Brown, and Mangalam 1971, p. 134)

This hypothesis is supported by the findings that fewer women than men (1) want to move to live in a different place, (2) want to return to the mountains, (3) want to be buried in the mountains, and (4) want to return to the mountains for retirement (Schwarzweller, Brown, and Mangalam 1971, pp. 140–41). They suspect that women see the amenities of urban life as a means to escape an earlier life that offered them little.

Women's greater alienation from the mountains, however, is not tempered by greater social affiliation or interaction with native Ohioans in the cities. Although the women had many non-Appalachian acquaintances, more than twice as many women as men did "not count any native of the urban areas as a 'close friend' with whom they meet in each other's homes" (Schwarzweller, Brown, and Mangalam 1971, p. 134). Because of their social isolation from those in the cities and their apparent desire not to return to the mountains, Appalachian women are caught between two cultures. They lack the social and emotional support needed to reduce the strains of the adjustment process, to ease their way into the opportunities offered by the urban environment, and to maintain the cultural contacts necessary for self-identity.

Appalachian culture provided ideal, acceptable roles for Appalachian mountain women. Roles that were appropriate in the mountain culture, however, are changing in urban areas. Although attitudes toward women's roles apparently are slow to change, economic and marital circumstances have necessitated changes in behavior.

The Appalachian patriarchal family structure has placed women in a subordinate role in the family. In urban areas, marital conflicts may occur because more responsibilities are placed on women in urban areas. Apparently, however, attitudes about Appalachian women's status are becoming more liberal among second-generation women and men; fewer of these individuals than of first-generation Appalachian migrants believe that men should have authority over women.

METHODOLOGY

We use the Davidson and Gordon model of the effect of ethnicity on gender roles to determine the influence on gender roles of self-identification with the Appalachian region, the existence of a cultural community, and the place of the group in the stratification system.

Data Source and Sample Size

This study uses data that James Brown (1950, cited by Schwarzweller, Brown, and Mangalam 1971) and Virginia McCoy collected in 1979 and 1982, which replicates data collected by Schwarzweller et al. in 1961–1963. The original study population consisted of 39 families living in three isolated communities, pseudonymously called Beech Creek. The 1982 data set includes all migrants from Beech Creek who were living and could be located in 1982. In 1962 the sample size was 140 migrants, including 71 women. In 1982 the sample size was 126, including 64 women (see Table 4.1). The 1962 and 1982 data sets contain data on the same individuals, excluding those who had died by 1982. Although we had only a small sample when conducting the regression analysis for women's roles, we took the appropriate steps to detect skewness, multicollinearity, normality, and measurement error (Tabachnick and Fidell 1983).

Operational Definitions

We tested the Davidson and Gordon model using the following operational definitions for self-identification, cultural community, and stratification.

Self-Identification Variables

Four variables were used as indicators of self-identification with Appalachian culture in the 1962 and 1982 data sets:

1. "Where do you feel is home?" (Kentucky, 0; any urban area/outside Kentucky, 1)
2. "How long until you felt this area was your home?" (more than one year, 0; one year or less, 1)

Table 4.1
Selected Variables, 1962, 1982

	1962		1982	
	All $N = 140$	Women $N = 71$	All $N = 126$	Women $N = 64$
Self-Identification				
Where do you feel is "home"?				
Kentucky (0)	55.7	52.1	23.3	15.6
Urban area (1)	44.3	47.9	76.7	84.4
How long until you felt at home?				
One year or less (1)	34.3	62.0	15.9	18.5
More than one year	65.7	38.0	84.1	81.5
Retirement location preference				
Kentucky (0)	41.4	38.0	18.9	23.4
Urban area (1)	58.6	62.0	81.1	76.6
Burial preference				
Kentucky (0)	54.3	52.1	29.5	23.4
Urban area (1)	45.7	47.9	70.5	76.6
Cultural Community				
Reason for moving				
Career or other (0)	—	—	44.4	64.6
Family (1)	—	—	55.6	35.4
Number families already there	2.9	1.9	—	—
Visiting Kentucky				
Yes (0)	67.1	66.2	47.6	44.6
No (1)	32.1	33.8	52.4	55.4
Number visits to Kentucky	1.4	1.4	3.1	3.4
Number native families	2.5	2.0	5.3	5.2
Stratification				
Income				
< $2,999	28.7	31.0	0.0	0.0
$3,000–$3,999	18.0	21.1	0.8	1.5
$4,000–$4,999	12.9	11.3	3.2	1.5
$5,000–$5,999	11.5	7.0	3.2	3.1
$6,000–$6,999	14.4	15.5	0.8	3.1
$7,000–$7,999	10.1	7.0	2.4	4.6
$8,000–$8,999	4.3 (+)	7.0 (+)	2.4	4.6
$9,000–$12,999	—	—	9.4	13.8
$13,000–$16,999	—	—	8.8	7.7
$17,000–$20,999	—	—	23.1	16.9
$21,000–$24,999	—	—	21.5	16.9
$25,000 and over	—	—	10.4	12.3

Table 4.1 continued

	1962		1982	
	All $N = 140$	Women $N = 71$	All $N = 126$	Women $N = 64$
Stratification continued				
Occupation				
White-collar	14.3	11.3	11.9	15.4
Blue-collar	28.6	12.7	49.2	33.8
Farmer	14.3	0.0	1.6	3.1
Homemaker	37.9	73.2	*	*
No main type of work/ retired/disabled	5.0	2.8	37.3	47.7
Power				
How are east Kentuckians treated here?				
All right (0)	84.3	83.1	95.2	95.4
Badly (1)	15.8	26.9	4.8	4.6

*Homemaker combined with no main type of work in 1982.

3. "Where do you prefer to live when you are too old to work?"
   (Kentucky, 0; any urban area/outside Kentucky, 1)

4. "Where do you prefer to be buried?" (Kentucky, 0; any urban
   area/outside Kentucky, 1)

Cultural Community Variables

We used the following variables as indicators of the presence of a
cultural community in the urban area where the respondent currently
lived:

1. We constructed this variable from two questions in the 1982
   data set: "What was the reason for moving (for any move after
   respondent had left eastern Kentucky) for any of seven
   moves?" If any move was made for "family-related reasons,"
   we coded it 1; all other reasons, including those for career, were
   coded 0. Moving for a family-related reason is more indicative
   of a cultural community than moving for any other reason.

2. The above question was unavailable in 1962; the closest
   question in the 1962 data set was, "How many families (close
   or distant relatives, friends, or acquaintances) did you know
   who already lived there?"

3. "Do you visit in Eastern Kentucky?" (yes, 1; no, 0)

4. Number of visits to Kentucky in the past 12 months.

5. "How many natives (of this area) do you know well enough to visit in each others' homes?"

Stratification Variables

1. We measured family income levels as follows: in 1962, income was categorized by thousand-dollar intervals, from below $1,000 to $8,000 or more. In 1982, it was categorized to correspond to the 1962 data set up to $8,999; after that level, it was collected by $4,000 intervals to $25,000, and then by $5,000 intervals to $70,000 or more.
2. Occupational level was collected in the 1962 data set by broad categories. To maintain comparability between the two data sets, we coded the 1982 variable using the same categories by status in this order: white-collar, blue-collar, farmer, homemaker, no main type of work/retired/disabled.
3. We measured perception of power in the community with the question, "How are eastern Kentuckians treated here?" (all right, 0; badly, 1) The respondent's perception of suffering discrimination indicates a sense of powerlessness.

Dependent Variable

We constructed the dependent variable from two questions, asking the respondent, "Is there anything in your life that you would have done differently?" First and second choices were elicited. The responses are categorized as school, religious, moral, financial, career, marriage, or none. If either of the two choices was school, career, or marriage, we coded them 1; other choices were coded 0. We believe that the choices coded 1 indicated a nontraditional role in regard to school, career, or marriage. Even though traditional roles might involve school or marriage, selection of these items might indicate a desire for a nontraditional role or a change from the current; 75 percent of women respondents in 1962 held traditional roles (Schwarzweller, Brown, and Mangalam 1971, pp. 142–43).

RESULTS

Identification with Appalachian culture was greater in 1962 than in 1982, especially for women. The 1962 data showed that slightly more than half the migrants identified with Kentucky in all the self-identification indicators except their preference for a retirement location; 58.6 percent preferred the urban area, and 41.4 percent preferred Kentucky. In 1982 the preference clearly shifted toward the urban areas, except for the respondents' recollection of the length of their period of adjustment to the urban area. A greater proportion of migrants recalled that adjustment took more than one year (84% in 1982 compared to 66% in 1962). This apparent discrepancy may reflect their adjustment to several different urban areas rather than to the one in which they currently lived. The respondents' greater identification with Kentucky in 1962 indicates a stronger identification with the Appalachian region, particularly eastern Kentucky. The shift in 1982 away from identification with Kentucky and toward identification with the urban area may indicate the respondents' integration into the urban area and loss of Appalachian identity.

We assessed the presence of a cultural community in the urban area by the degree to which visits were made primarily with eastern Kentucky family and friends and with family or friends in the urban area. The 1962 pattern reveals a clear preference for visits in eastern Kentucky. Half of the sample did not know any families when they moved to the area.

Of the remaining half, 15 percent knew one or two families, 10 percent knew up to four families, and the remainder knew up to eight families. Sixty-seven percent visited in eastern Kentucky, with a mean of 1.4 visits. The 1962 sample visited with few native northern families in their homes, with a mean of 2.5 visits.

The 1982 pattern is less definitive than the 1962 pattern. A greater proportion of families moved around in urban locations for family reasons than for other reasons; slightly more than half had *not* visited in eastern Kentucky during the previous year.

The pattern of stratification as shown by income and occupation data reveals a lower level than in the general population of cities such as Cincinnati. A greater number of Appalachians hold blue-collar jobs; a greater number maintain traditional jobs, working at home; fewer Appalachians hold white-collar jobs. Between 1962 and 1982, migrants became even more entrenched in the blue-collar work force. The indicator for power, a proxy for perception of discrimination, shows clearly that few persons felt mistreated.

Women's self-identification indicators show patterns similar to those for the group as a whole, except that the changes between 1962 and 1982 are more dramatic. In 1962, 47.9 percent of women felt that their home was in the city; by 1982, 84.4 percent did so. In 1962, 38 percent of the women responded that it took longer than a year to begin to feel at home in the city; in 1982, this proportion increased dramatically to 81.5

percent. A greater proportion of women wanted to be buried in the urban area and preferred the urban area for retirement in 1982 than in 1962.

The cultural community variables show that fewer women visited in Kentucky in 1982 than in 1962, but the mean number of visits increased slightly. The number of native families whom the women knew well enough to visit also increased.

The stratification indicators show an interesting pattern for women. Women's improvement in occupational status is indicated by the increase in the proportion holding white-collar jobs and by the increase in the proportion holding blue-collar jobs in 1982.

The indicator for power, a proxy for discrimination, shows that few women felt that they were treated badly in the city, either as newcomers in 1962 or in 1982.

Table 4.2
Logistic Regression Results: Effect of Ethnicity on Gender Roles

Theoretical Variables	Parameter Estimates		
	1982 All	1982 Six-Variable Model All	1982 Six-Variable Model Women
Self-Identification			
Home	0.4460	0.4127	0.0756
Homelong	-0.2564		
Retire	0.6666		
Bury	-1.2629*	-0.8345	-0.1882
Cultural Community			
Moving reasons	-0.3733		
Visit Kentucky	-0.0491	-0.0814	0.4554
Number visits	-0.0386		
Number natives	0.0276	0.0280	-0.0174
Stratification			
Income	-0.0016		
Occupation	-0.0070	-0.0069	-0.0057
Discrimination	0.5372	0.6130	0.4921
Intercept	0.5251	0.3166	0.1009

$* p < 0.05$

In determining the effect of ethnicity on gender roles, we examined only 1982 data. The dependent variable (role) in the 1962 data showed too little variation to permit a meaningful analysis for that year; only 14 percent of women were nontraditional in that they had considered changing to a nontraditional role. In 1982 the dependent variable showed that 50.8 percent of women would choose nontraditional roles and 49.2 percent would choose traditional roles; 50 percent would choose each category when given the option.

We performed logistic regression analysis on the configuration of theoretical variables for the total sample to determine whether the Davidson and Gordon model explained choosing a change in roles (see Table 4.2). This analysis resulted in an insignificant model (chi-square = 9.864; p = 0.6). In addition, we selected two variables to represent each theoretical concept and logistic analysis that we applied. This process also resulted in an insignificant model (chi-square = 5.219; p = 0.5). Because of the small number of cases, we tested only the six-variable model for women. The results were insignificant (chi-square = 1.966; p = 0.9).

DISCUSSION

The traditional roles of Appalachian women appear to be changing. Between 1962 and 1982 the proportion of women who would consider a nontraditional role increased considerably, although in 1982 only half of the women would do so. Substantial changes in occupational status are evident in the decrease in the number of women working in the home and in the increase in the proportion of women in white-collar occupations. The unique place of Appalachians in the stratification system as blue-collar workers may make them noteworthy for their identification with the working class, although a sizable proportion of women are in white-collar occupations.

There is also evidence that the Appalachians in the study (particularly the women) are showing a greater affinity for the city and less affinity for their "homes" in eastern Kentucky.

Although the Davidson and Gordon model did not appear to influence changes in gender role, this result may be attributed to limitations due to the small sample size or limitations in the operational definitions of the concepts, especially the dependent variable, gender role.

Role changes in Appalachian culture may result in greater opportunities for Appalachian women in urban areas, especially unmarried women who may be less confined by the patriarchal family structure. Married women, on the other hand, may begin to experience more power in the family unit. As discussed above, however, conflicts that accompany the change in authority are likely to produce some instability.

Changes for Appalachian women that accompany adjustment to urban areas may create role conflicts. Many women are caught between two worlds: they are different from those they left behind in the mountains and different from other urban women. This situation may create a bicultural identity for some women, who may retain part of the mountain culture while adopting parts of the urban culture that seem appropriate in the city.

II

Health and Environmental Issues

5

Urban Appalachian Health Concerns
Phillip J. Obermiller and Robert W. Oldendick

Clarity of communication between patients and health care providers is tempered by a number of variables, including the ethnic background and the cultural expectations of those who are served. Whereas many health care professionals have been made aware of the special health concerns of Asians, Hispanics, and blacks, other cultural groups are not identified as easily, nor is consciousness of their culture as widespread. This is particularly true of Appalachian migrants.

Medical anthropologist John Friedl points out:

Limited education created a serious barrier in communication between an [urban] Appalachian patient and a health care professional. Poor communication can quite obviously detract from the quality of care received, and in many cases can lead to alienation that ultimately drives the patient away from the health care system. (1983, p. 190)

Friedl notes, however, that the problem of education is mutual:

The professional jargon and middle-class educated speech patterns used by health care providers create a cultural gap between them and many of their clients, including Appalachian migrants....Among recent migrants, different names for health problems are often used which are not understood by non-Appalachian physicians, nurses, and other professionals. Even accents and speech patterns can create serious barriers to effective personal interaction in the health care setting. (1983, p. 205)

Now that large numbers of first- and second-generation Appalachian migrants live in major metropolitan areas of the United States, urban health care providers have a greater need for accurate information about the cultural background and the special health concerns of this group.

Such practical knowledge can enhance communication between patient and provider and can increase the effectiveness of diagnostic procedures, treatment compliance, and patient education.

In this chapter, we examine the medical beliefs and practices of urban Appalachians and contrast them with those of two other urban groups: blacks and non-Appalachian whites. We begin by examining previous studies of urban Appalachian medical beliefs and practices. Using a comparative model, we examine (1) the three groups' concerns about six major health risks; (2) their smoking, diet, and exercise behaviors; and (3) their beliefs about the causes of good health and illness. We analyze these findings in the discussion and will conclude with some specific suggestions for serving urban Appalachian patients more effectively.

PREVIOUS STUDIES

Although health issues and service strategies in the Appalachian region are reasonably well documented (Appalachian Center 1986; Couto 1978, 1983; C. H. Hamilton 1962; Loof 1971; Obermiller and Oldendick 1987; Pearsall 1960), substantially less is known about the health problems and the accessibility of medical services for urban Appalachians. Much of the literature on urban Appalachian health concerns is quite dated (Porter 1961, 1963a, 1963b; Powles 1964; Watkins 1973), is obscure, or appears as incidental sections of larger reports (Philliber 1981b). The key contributions to the literature are studies by Watkins (1973) and Friedl (1978, 1983).

Virginia McCoy Watkins (1973) notes the key roles of home remedies, folk medical practices, and faith healing in the migrants' background. Modern medicine is not unknown in the mountains but is relatively difficult to obtain. Few opportunities for nutritional education or for preventive health care measures are available. Watkins points out that in the mountains health care generally is sought and provided on a crisis basis. Medical procedures under emergency conditions are drastic, impersonal, and frequently ineffective; this unfortunate situation, usually accompanied by many unfamiliar bureaucratic forms and procedures, fosters a fear and a suspicion of health care providers that Appalachians bring with them into urban environments.

In a study of health problems faced by Appalachians, John Friedl (1978) interviewed 51 providers and 106 Appalachian migrant families in Columbus, Ohio, about health-related topics. His findings are consistent with Watkins's in that the rural health care experiences of

Appalachian migrants influence their expectations of urban health care providers. The physician in the mountains has fewer staff resources and therefore more direct contact with the patient. Because of cost and travel time, referrals to distant specialists are rare; for similar reasons the mountain physician is more likely to attempt a "one-shot" cure than a series of treatments, and drugs are distributed more frequently at the time of treatment than by prescription. Third-party payments are less typical in rural areas, so fees are lower and payment schedules are more flexible. The sharp contrast between styles of health care service in rural and in urban settings often leads to confusion, distrust, and negative stereotypes on the part of both the Appalachian migrant and the urban medical provider.

THE CURRENT STUDY

Whereas previous studies focus on Appalachian migrants and their interaction with urban health care systems, this study compares the health concerns and behaviors of urban Appalachians with those of their black and non-Appalachian white counterparts in the city. The cultural characteristics of urban Appalachians are maintained through extended family networks, tightly knit occupational and residential patterns, and visits to their counties of origin. Migration from the region peaked 30 years ago, however, and the migrants' children and grandchildren have grown up in urban neighborhoods. Therefore, this study explores the differences between contemporary urban Appalachians and other urban groups in regard to health concerns, behaviors, and beliefs.

The data employed in this study were collected as part of the fall 1987 Greater Cincinnati Survey, a random-digit-dialed telephone survey of adult residents of Hamilton County, Ohio. As part of this survey, interviews were conducted with 512 residents of the city of Cincinnati, who were asked a series of questions about their health, health-related concerns, and health care behaviors.

Questions concerning the birthplaces of the respondent and the respondent's parents were not included in this survey, so we could not use this method for determining Appalachian origin. Therefore, in conducting this secondary analysis, we were forced to use a different approach in identifying Appalachian respondents. The validity of this approach is crucial for the analyses presented here, so we will describe our methods in some detail.

The residential clustering of Appalachian migrants in urban neighborhoods has been well documented (Fowler 1981; Fowler and

Davies 1972; Maloney 1985; Philliber 1981b). We elected to follow the typology of the social areas of Cincinnati developed by Maloney (1985) for the city's Human Relations Commission. In his classification, Maloney develops objective criteria for classifying census tracts (aggregated into neighborhoods) as predominantly black, Appalachian, or white.

Neighborhoods are designated as black if the black population exceeds the city average of 35.4 percent. This measure is conservative because neighborhoods so designated are, on the average, 75.8 percent black (Maloney 1985).

Because Appalachians are not readily identifiable from census data, Maloney establishes seven criteria for classifying a Cincinnati neighborhood as Appalachian: (1) more than 19.14 percent of the families are below poverty level; (2) fewer than 35.36 percent of the residents are black; (3) fewer than 51 percent of the residents age 25 and older are high school graduates; (4) more than 18 percent of the out-of-school population between ages 16 and 19 are not high school graduates; (5) more than 12.6 percent of the population between ages 16 and 19 are jobless; (6) more than 34.4 percent of the population are service, semiskilled, or unskilled workers; and (7) family size averages more than 3.19 persons.

Using the standards set forth above, Maloney classified 16 Cincinnati neighborhoods as black, 9 as Appalachian, and the remaining 23 as white.

Because a question about race was asked of these respondents, the data for blacks allow us to test these procedures. Among those who were identified as black on the basis of their residence, 74 percent were black and 26 percent were white. Similarly, the census location categorized 62 percent of those who actually were black as black and 93 percent of those who actually were white as white. Although these procedures produce some misclassifications, a significant overlap exists between reported race and the race designated on the basis of this classification scheme.

We refined this measure further by taking those blacks who were classified as "other whites" on the basis of census tracts and placing them into the black category, and by transferring those whites who were classified as black into the "other white" category. As a result of this adjustment, everyone classified in the black category is black; the Appalachian category contains respondents living in tracts that are classified as Appalachian (including some non-Appalachian whites and some blacks); and the "other white" category consists entirely of white respondents, including those white Appalachians who live in the city in tracts not classified as Appalachian. The effect of these misclassifications is conservative: differences that exist between Appalachians and other whites may be muted because the Appalachian classification is not pure and because some Appalachians are classified as "other whites."

We recognize the hazards involved in attempting to infer individual characteristics on the basis of aggregate statistics. Still, we believe that our approach is the most reasonable method for examining this question in view of what is known about the residential clustering of Appalachians, the results obtained by using this approach with black respondents, our ability to refine this measure to some extent, and the lack of any other means for identifying Appalachian respondents with these data. As mentioned previously, the effect of this inability to identify Appalachians more precisely is moderation of the differences between Appalachians and other groups; the results reported here should be interpreted with this fact in mind.

Of the 512 city residents interviewed, 146 (28.5%) were black, 75 (14.6%) were categorized as Appalachian, and 291 (56.9%) were designated as "other whites." The proportions of these groups in the city's population are consistent with those found in earlier studies; similarly, the proportion of Appalachians identified as black in this study coincides with that found in previous research (Community Chest and Council of the Cincinnati Area 1983; Philliber and Obermiller 1982).

FINDINGS

Table 5.1 presents a comparison of black, Appalachian, and non-Appalachian white respondents' concerns about six specific health risks and about overall health. We found significant differences in concern on each of the specific risks (with the exception of diabetes) and in concern for overall health. Blacks and Appalachians show similar concerns about the risks of heart attack, stroke, emotional or mental illness, or serious accidental injury. Non-Appalachian whites are generally less concerned about these problems. Blacks and Appalachians differ in their concern about cancer; about 38 percent of blacks are extremely concerned, compared with 21 percent of Appalachians and 18 percent of non-Appalachian whites. Concerns about overall health also differentiate the three groups. Blacks show the highest percentage of respondents who are extremely concerned about their overall health (28%), while only 8 percent of non-Appalachian whites express such extreme concern. The percentage of Appalachians extremely concerned about their overall health (16%) falls between these two groups.

Table 5.1
Comparison of Concerns of Blacks, Appalachians, and Whites in Cincinnati about Selected Health-Related Topics, 1987

	Blacks %	Appalachians %	Whites %
Cancer*			
Extremely concerned	37.7	21.3	18.3
Not too concerned	25.9	23.5	34.5
Heart Attack*			
Extremely concerned	21.9	25.3	11.9
Not too concerned	24.5	34.4	31.9
Diabetes			
Extremely concerned	13.5	9.7	11.4
Not too concerned	39.7	49.7	53.9
Stroke*			
Extremely concerned	16.0	20.0	10.0
Not too concerned	25.1	32.3	49.1
Emotional or Mental Illness*			
Extremely concerned	13.6	11.3	6.1
Not too concerned	53.0	46.9	66.3
Serious Accidental Injury*			
Extremely concerned	20.4	22.7	8.0
Not too concerned	22.6	22.0	42.8
Overall Health*			
Extremely concerned	27.6	16.0	7.8
Not too concerned	12.5	16.6	28.4

* Indicates $p < 0.001$.

Overall, blacks and Appalachians exhibit more concern about a variety of health risks than do non-Appalachian whites. These two groups, however, differ on their concern about cancer and about their overall health; a higher percentage of blacks than of Appalachians is extremely concerned about these factors.

When questioned about beliefs and practices regarding diet and exercise, each of the three groups expresses approximately the same opinions and behaviors (see Table 5.2). More people in the sample believe in the importance of exercise than actually exercise weekly. The same is true of diet, but the gap between belief and practice is larger for diet than for exercise.

Although Table 5.2 shows that more than three quarters of each group associate smoking with cancer and heart disease, more than two thirds of the Appalachian respondents are currently smokers, as compared with fewer than one third of the black and the other white cohorts.

Table 5.2
Comparison of the Opinions and Behaviors of Blacks, Appalachians, and Whites in Cincinnati about Selected Health Issues, 1987

	Blacks %	Appalachians %	Whites %
Smoking			
Associates smoking with cancer or heart disease	90.9	75.9	86.0
Respondent currently is a smoker*	32.0	68.7	30.3
Exercise			
Believes strongly in the importance of exercise	80.4	63.6	68.9
Respondent exercises at least four times a week	58.7	58.5	50.1
Diet			
Believes strongly in the importance of a balanced diet	81.7	85.7	81.9
Respondent almost always eats a balanced diet	23.0	10.6	24.6

* Indicates $p < 0.001$.

Table 5.3 presents data on the respondents' beliefs about the causes of good and bad health. A large proportion of each group believes in the influence of self-care; smaller but substantial numbers believe that their health is influenced by heredity, family, and friends. Fewer still attribute their good health to luck or their poor health to God; very few believe that illness is a result of failure by the physician.

Despite overall similarities in beliefs about the causes of good or bad health, some interesting divergences occur among the three groups. Substantially more Appalachians and blacks than non-Appalachian whites believe that illness is caused by God. Appalachians are least likely to believe that one can avoid illness by taking good care of oneself, while other whites show the highest percentage of those who believe that relationships with family and friends affect one's health.

Table 5.3
Comparison of the Beliefs of Blacks, Appalachians, and Whites in Cincinnati about Various Influences on Health, 1987

	Blacks %	Appalachians %	Whites %
Influence of Heredity			
Believes strongly that genetic inheritance influences health	38.9	36.6	48.5
Influence of Luck			
Believes that good health is a matter of good luck	19.5	26.5	19.7
Influence of Family and Friends*			
Believes that relationships with family and friends affect respondent's health	35.7	39.2	42.9
Influence of God*			
Believes that illness is caused by God	29.4	22.0	6.2
Influence of Self-Care*			
Believes that one can avoid illness by taking good care of self	87.7	64.4	81.1
Influence of Physician			
Believes that illness is due to failure on doctor's part	0.3	5.8	2.7

* indicates $p < 0.001$.

DISCUSSION

Although the process of assimilation apparently has reduced the importance of the Appalachians' rural background and migration experiences, health care professionals would be remiss to ignore their Appalachian patients' heritage. The evidence presented above shows that urban Appalachians cannot be categorized readily by either class or race.

Blacks and non-Appalachian whites cite cancer as their primary health concern, followed by heart disease. Among Appalachians, however, heart disease is the primary concern, followed by accidental injury and cancer. A much lower percentage of non-Appalachian whites than of either Appalachians or blacks is concerned about accidental injury.

Appalachians' concerns about heart disease can be linked to smoking, which we discuss below. The concern about accidental injury may be related to the fact that many Appalachians have experienced the perils of working in the central Appalachian coalfields and driving on dangerous mountain roads. In addition, urban Appalachian workers (as well as blacks) frequently are employed in manufacturing and service jobs with high incidences of occupational hazards. The relatively low concern about cancer can be attributed to the deceptively low incidence of certain cancers in the Appalachian region.

The data show that urban Appalachians are similar to other city residents in their knowledge about the consequences of smoking, regular exercise, and proper nutrition. Yet they are more than twice as likely to be smokers as the black or the other white respondents. Most urban Appalachians have roots in a rural region whose main cash crop is tobacco; the use of tobacco products not only is socially acceptable among mountain men and women but also is widely perceived as critical for economic survival.

The urban Appalachians are less likely than other whites to believe that genetic inheritance strongly influences overall health; they are more likely to believe that good health is a matter of luck and that illness is caused by God. These opinions can be associated with the fundamentalist religious beliefs typically found in the Appalachian region and throughout the rural South. Concepts of genetic mutation and inheritance are linked closely with arguments for human evolution, a scientific tenet that conflicts with literal interpretations of the Bible. Similarly, in fundamentalist belief, the hand of God is involved directly in human affairs, including punishment through illness and forgiveness through healing.

CONCLUSION

Although some urban Appalachians are now two and three generations removed from mountain life and the migration experience, it is premature to assume that assimilation has eliminated a particular cultural perspective from their health care concerns and needs. Alert health care providers can identify the urban Appalachian neighborhoods in their service areas. Informal screening techniques, such as asking where the patient's parents or grandparents used to live, can confirm Appalachian heritage.

A basic knowledge of Appalachian history and culture on the part of health care professionals can do much to alleviate miscommunication, particularly in areas where scientific and religious assumptions come into conflict. Diagnosis can be expedited by understanding the occupational health hazards typically faced by Appalachian workers; many black lung victims move to urban neighborhoods after they become disabled. Educational programs aimed at stopping or reducing smoking, when presented properly, can have a positive effect on urban Appalachians' well-being.

As with other groups of health care consumers, adding a cultural perspective to medical competence can greatly enhance medical services to urban Appalachians.

6

Health Education Strategies
for Urban Blacks and Appalachians

Phillip J. Obermiller and Walter S. Handy, Jr.

It has now become almost axiomatic that future gains in longevity among all members of the U.S. population will be achieved through changes in how we live. Medical science continues to make important technological advances in methods to prolong the lives of those who are most ill and infirm. These costly advances, however, are unlikely to be affordable for most Americans and will not substantially increase the longevity of those who do receive treatment. The alternative, promoting health throughout the life spans of all citizens, promises to be much more effective for the majority of people.

In this chapter, we regard health promotion as any combination of health education, environmental safeguards, and social reinforcement for behavior conducive to good health (Levin 1987; Terris 1986). Health promotion can affect individual, group, and community behaviors and can be conducted both through professionally designed programs and through grass-roots efforts. In short, everybody can participate in health promotion and everyone can benefit from it (Greene et al. 1980).

Moreover, some segments of the population experience higher health risks than others. Age is one key factor; youth are more susceptible to alcohol abuse, whereas seniors are more likely to experience hypertension (Damberg 1986; Minkler and Passick 1986). Socioeconomic status is another important indicator; people with more education and higher incomes are more likely to avoid smoking, to wear seat belts, and to exercise than less educated, financially less well-off individuals (Labonte 1986; Syme and Berkman 1976). Other major influences on health are racial and ethnic differences (Fruend 1984; Galli, Greenberg, and Tobin 1987; Nugent et al. 1988). Obesity, for instance, is a more serious problem among blacks than among whites; as one might expect, pneumoconiosis is more prevalent among workers from the Appalachian region than from other areas of the country.

PURPOSE

Clearly, then, effective health education must take into account the heterogeneity of the population in which it is to be offered. Specific cultural and social differences must be considered in the design and implementation of health promotion programs.

Blacks and Appalachians are two minority groups that have sizable populations in most midwestern cities. In this chapter, we present a case study that examines the black, Appalachian, and non-Appalachian white population in a single midwestern metropolis. We examine the health status, health maintenance activities, and sources of health and wellness information for each of these three groups in order to discern patterns of behavior that would form the basis for an effective health promotion program. Our conclusions result in recommendations for tailoring health promotion activities to the needs of urban blacks and Appalachians.

THE DATA

The demographic characteristics of urban Appalachians were presented in the earlier chapters of this book, and the health literature on the group was reviewed in Chapter 5. In this chapter, we use data obtained from the 1989 Greater Cincinnati Survey, a random-digit-dialed survey that included 175 black, 160 Appalachian white, and 575 non-Appalachian white residents of the city of Cincinnati. Black Appalachians are included in the black group because in the United States race dominates ethnicity as a social characteristic. *Urban Appalachians* are defined as having been born or having a parent who was born in one of the federally designated Appalachian counties.

FINDINGS

In Table 6.1 the concern about overall health is shown for each of the three groups. Blacks show significantly more concern about their health than do the two white groups. A large difference also exists in the utilization of emergency room services, according to the data in Table 6.2. Blacks are by far the most likely of the groups to use emergency care; Appalachians are the least likely.

Table 6.1
Comparison of the Concerns of Whites, Appalachians, and Blacks in Cincinnati about Their Overall Health, 1989

	Whites		Appalachians		Blacks	
	%	N	%	N	%	N
Extremely concerned	16.4	36	20.9	17	26.3	34
Very concerned	30.2	66	25.5	20	38.6	50
Somewhat concerned	28.8	63	30.6	24	12.4	16
Not too concerned	24.7	54	23.0	18	22.7	29

$p < 0.001$.

Table 6.2
Number of Trips to an Emergency Room in the Past Four or Five Months: Whites, Appalachians, and Blacks in Cincinnati, 1989

	Whites		Appalachians		Blacks	
	%	N	%	N	%	N
1	18.2	40	13.1	10	22.3	29
2	3.3	7	5.2	4	5.7	7
3	1.1	3	—	—	3.6	5
4	—	—	—	—	3.5	5
5	—	—	—	—	0.5	1
6 or more	0.3	1	0.8	1	2.5	3
None	77.1	169	81.0	64	61.8	80

$p < 0.001$.

It would seem reasonable to conclude that emergency services often are required when routine prevention and treatment are either postponed or omitted altogether. Table 6.3, however, shows that emergency care does not necessarily escalate with lack of physical checkups. On the contrary, the three groups have about the same relative number of physicals, although blacks have the most and Appalachians have the least in absolute numbers.

Table 6.3
Whites, Appalachians, and Blacks in Cincinnati Who Have Had a Physical Checkup in the Past Four or Five Months, 1989

	Whites		Appalachians		Blacks	
	%	N	%	N	%	N
Have had a physical	33.4	73	30.5	24	41.4	53
Have not had a physical	66.6	146	69.5	55	58.6	75

64 *From Mountain to Metropolis*

The same finding is corroborated by the data in Table 6.4, which shows doctor visits for each of the three groups. Non-Appalachian whites had the fewest doctor's appointments; blacks had the most. The Appalachians form a middle group, but some apparently experienced illnesses severe enough to require frequent office visits over a relatively short period.

Table 6.4
Number of Times Respondent Has Seen a Doctor for Reasons Other Than an Emergency or a Physical in the Past Four or Five Months: Whites, Appalachians, and Blacks in Cincinnati, 1989

	Whites		Appalachians		Blacks	
	%	N	%	N	%	N
1	11.8	26	13.8	11	17.0	22
2	7.7	17	9.7	8	10.2	13
3	8.8	19	0.9	1	4.1	5
4	3.3	7	1.5	1	4.1	5
5	6.5	14	0.5	1	1.8	2
6 or more	7.9	17	17.0	13	5.1	6
None	54.1	118	56.6	45	57.6	74

$p < 0.001.$

Table 6.5 shows that the two white groups are hospitalized at a significantly lower rate than the black group. Of the three groups, blacks are most likely to be hospitalized, and the length of hospitalization is longer for blacks and Appalachians once they are admitted. The indication that urban Appalachians may suffer from severe illnesses is borne out in the length of their hospital stays.

Table 6.5
Number of Days Respondent Has Spent in a Hospital in the Past Four or Five Months: Whites, Appalachians, and Blacks in Cincinnati, 1989

	Whites		Appalachians		Blacks	
	%	N	%	N	%	N
1 or 2	2.1	5	—	—	0.4	1
3 or 5	1.2	3	2.7	2	2.1	3
6 or 9	—	—	—	—	5.5	7
10 or 14	2.0	4	—	—	1.0	1
15 or 19	—	—	0.8	1	—	—
20 or more	—	—	1.5	1	2.0	3
None	94.6	207	95.0	75	89.0	115

$p < 0.001.$

In Table 6.6 the data show that significantly more Appalachians are out of both the labor force and the school population than blacks or other whites. This finding may account for their low incidence of absences from work or school (16%), as compared with that for non-Appalachian whites (26.5%) and blacks (24.7%).

Table 6.6
Number of Days Missed at School or Work Because of Health Problems: Whites, Appalachians, and Blacks in Cincinnati, 1989

	Whites		Appalachians		Blacks	
	%	N	%	N	%	N
1 or 2	16.1	35	6.4	5	12.7	16
3 or 5	4.6	10	8.3	6	3.3	4
6 or 9	2.0	4	—	—	6.5	8
10 to 14	0.8	2	—	—	0.4	1
15 to 19	0.8	2	—	—	—	—
20 or more	2.2	5	1.3	1	1.8	2
None	54.5	119	38.8	30	52.9	68
Not in school or work	18.9	41	45.2	35	22.4	29

$p < 0.001$.

Tables 6.7, 6.8, and 6.9 show the sources of personal health information used by the three groups. The data indicate clear differences. The Appalachians obtain most of their health knowledge from doctors, nurses, relatives, and the media; they receive relatively little from health care facilities, friends, or churches. Blacks rely heavily on health

Table 6.7
Sources of Personal Health Information for Whites in Cincinnati, 1989

	Great Deal		Some		Not Much		None	
	%	N	%	N	%	N	%	N
Doctors	35.0	77	28.5	62	23.0	50	13.6	30
Nurses	16.2	35	21.5	47	26.6	58	35.8	78
Television/radio	14.5	31	41.2	89	20.3	44	24.1	52
Newspapers/ magazines	19.2	42	44.6	97	15.2	33	21.0	46
Hospitals/clinics	5.1	11	18.7	41	22.1	48	54.0	118
Churches	1.0	2	7.5	16	13.6	30	77.9	170
Relatives	15.6	34	31.1	68	15.6	34	37.7	82
Friends	10.8	24	30.3	66	15.4	34	43.5	95

Table 6.8
Sources of Personal Health Information for Appalachians in Cincinnati, 1989

	Great Deal		Some		Not Much		None	
	%	N	%	N	%	N	%	N
Doctors	41.5	33	28.2	22	3.3	3	27.0	21
Nurses	27.5	22	26.5	21	14.0	11	31.9	25
Television/radio	24.5	19	29.1	23	17.8	14	28.6	23
Newspapers/ magazines	20.0	16	44.6	35	13.1	10	22.3	18
Hospitals/clinics	11.9	9	37.4	30	10.8	9	40.0	32
Churches	0.5	1	9.8	8	9.8	8	79.8	63
Relatives	24.8	20	19.7	16	6.5	5	49.0	39
Friends	7.9	6	29.1	23	14.3	11	48.8	39

Table 6.9
Sources of Personal Health Information for Blacks in Cincinnati, 1989

	Great Deal		Some		Not Much		None	
	%	N	%	N	%	N	%	N
Doctors	49.4	64	20.5	26	11.4	15	18.7	24
Nurses	18.5	24	23.6	30	17.6	23	40.3	52
Television/radio	31.4	40	38.0	49	16.9	22	13.6	18
Newspapers/ magazines	23.6	30	35.3	45	13.8	18	27.3	35
Hospitals/clinics	28.9	37	28.5	37	10.6	14	32.0	41
Churches	11.3	14	10.8	14	18.2	23	59.6	76
Relatives	20.5	26	34.7	45	20.4	26	24.4	31
Friends	11.9	15	39.8	51	20.5	26	27.9	36

professionals for their information, as well as on the media, health care facilities, and relatives. Although blacks are less likely to look to friends or to churches than to the other sources, they rely significantly more on their churches for health information than do the other two groups.

The sources of information for staying healthy (i.e., wellness) are compared for the three groups in Tables 6.10, 6.11, and 6.12. The three groups differ clearly as to sources of wellness information; within each group they differ as to the sources used for personal health information or wellness education. For information about staying healthy, Appalachians rely primarily on health professionals and the media and report progressively less reliance on health care institutions, relatives, friends, and churches. When Appalachians seek wellness education, they rely less on doctors and nurses and more on the media than when they are seeking personal health information.

Doctors are the primary sources of both personal health and wellness information in the black community; the media and health facilities follow closely. Blacks make relatively less use of nurses, relatives, churches, and friends, although in absolute numbers, they use even these sources extensively.

Table 6.10
Sources of Wellness Information for Whites in Cincinnati, 1989

	Great Deal		Some		Not Much		None	
	%	N	%	N	%	N	%	N
Doctors	23.8	52	32.9	72	23.8	52	19.4	43
Nurses	9.0	20	28.0	61	23.7	52	39.2	86
Television/ radio	21.7	47	44.9	98	13.1	29	20.4	44
Newspapers/ magazines	23.3	51	46.0	101	14.7	32	16.0	35
Hospitals/ clinics	7.0	15	20.3	44	21.8	48	50.9	111
Churches	1.0	2	8.6	19	13.8	30	76.6	167
Relatives	15.6	34	38.8	85	10.5	23	35.1	77
Friends	10.0	22	39.1	86	13.7	30	37.2	81

Table 6.11
Sources of Wellness Information for Appalachians in Cincinnati, 1989

	Great Deal		Some		Not Much		None	
	%	N	%	N	%	N	%	N
Doctors	26.0	21	31.3	25	13.4	11	29.3	23
Nurses	22.8	18	24.0	19	14.9	12	38.3	30
Television/radio	18.2	14	44.4	35	18.6	15	18.8	15
Newspapers/ magazines	18.4	15	42.7	34	15.6	12	23.3	18
Hospitals/clinics	14.0	11	21.1	17	20.1	16	44.8	36
Churches	0.5	1	5.2	4	11.7	9	82.7	65
Relatives	10.0	8	30.6	24	11.1	9	48.3	38
Friends	5.8	5	30.5	24	15.8	13	47.8	38

Table 6.12
Sources of Wellness Information for Blacks in Cincinnati, 1989

| | Great Deal | | Some | | Not Much | | None | |
	%	N	%	N	%	N	%	N
Doctors	48.9	62	28.1	36	9.	13	13.1	17
Nurses	22.2	28	34.3	44	14.8	19	28.7	36
Television/radio	38.6	49	31.9	40	19.2	24	10.3	13
Newspapers/								
magazines	28.2	36	38.9	49	14.5	18	18.4	23
Hospitals/clinics	33.1	42	22.6	29	19.3	24	25.1	32
Churches	13.2	17	16.5	21	27.7	35	42.6	54
Relatives	21.8	28	43.9	55	10.9	14	23.3	29
Friends	10.7	14	40.9	52	25.1	32	32.3	29

Non-Appalachian whites are the least likely of the three groups to seek wellness information from their physicians. For this group, radio, television, newspapers, and magazines are almost as important as doctors for wellness education. Relatively few members of this group look to health care facilities or churches for this type of information.

CONCLUSIONS AND RECOMMENDATIONS

The high levels of concern about health among blacks suggest that this group should be highly receptive to efforts at health education. Relatively lower levels of health concern in the white cohort should lead health educators to focus initially on motivational techniques. The fact that well over two fifths of both the Appalachians and the non-Appalachian whites were either extremely concerned or very concerned about their health should provide a sound basis for reaching the less health-conscious portions of those groups.

The heavy use of emergency services among blacks indicates a point of contact for health education. Hospitals and clinics might consider their emergency room waiting rooms as sites for some type of patient education. This strategy, however, would be much less effective for contacting members of the white cohorts because emergency service utilization among whites is low, particularly among Appalachians.

About three fifths of each group reported no physical checkup in the four or five months preceding the survey. In regard to health promotion, this area obviously requires emphasis. Increasing the use of regular physical checkups could benefit large numbers of all three groups; the Appalachians display the largest potential for health gains.

Physician contacts are high for blacks; this finding indicates blacks' relatively great need for health care as well as suggesting another important avenue for health education. Although relatively few Appalachians see doctors, those who do so see them quite often; this fact may signify a need for assistance in coping with chronic conditions.

Hospital stays are significantly higher for blacks than for the two white cohorts; once again, this finding indicates an opportunity for patient education at health care facilities. Appalachians report the fewest days of hospitalization but display a tendency to stay longer once hospitalized. Probably in those cases, they are seriously ill, and hospitalization has been delayed until well along in the course of the illness. These facts have obvious implications for health education: early diagnosis and intervention and treatment compliance should be emphasized for this group.

The large proportion of the Appalachian group that neither goes to work nor attends school suggests several possibilities. Some may be at home raising families; some may be school dropouts in their teens or early twenties; some may be older, retired persons; others may be unemployed workers. This heterogeneity calls for diversity in the approaches to health promotion in the urban Appalachian community. Most appropriate would be a multifaceted plan including, for example, substance abuse counseling, advice on stress reduction, information on children's health, and health programs for seniors.

Tables 6.7 through 6.12 provide a wealth of information on how to introduce health education programs into the three communities. Although doctors play a primary role for each group, clear differences emerge in the alternatives selected by each group for additional information on health care and wellness. Relatives rank comparatively high as information sources for Appalachians; churches maintain an important role in health education among blacks. The electronic media are more salient for blacks and Appalachians, whereas the print media are more important for non-Appalachian whites. Nurses are better potential sources of health education for the Appalachians than for blacks and other whites. Hospitals and clinics are more likely to be considered good sources of health information by blacks than by Appalachians or other whites. All three groups regard kinship networks as better sources of health care advice than friendship networks.

Important racial and ethnic differences must be taken into consideration in designing programs for health promotion in urban communities. In this chapter, we have pointed out those differences for urban blacks and Appalachians and have suggested useful approaches to health education based on those distinctions.

7

The Health Status of Children Living in Urban Appalachian Neighborhoods

M. Kathryn Brown and Phillip J. Obermiller

Outmigration has been a recognized phenomenon in the life of the Appalachian region for most of the twentieth century. Economic and sociocultural factors have combined to influence the movement of people into and out of Appalachia with increasing significance in the past 60 years (Brown and Hillery 1962; McCoy and Brown 1981; Obermiller and Oldendick 1987). As a result of the migration streams, multigenerational Appalachian families now constitute the majority population in many urban neighborhoods across the Midwest.

The social adjustment of Appalachian families moving to urban areas follows a familiar pattern: it focused initially on finding housing and employment, then on obtaining an education, and finally on deferred concerns such as health care. A growing body of literature examines the settlement and employment patterns and the educational attainment of urban Appalachian adults (Obermiller and Philliber 1987; Philliber 1981b; Philliber and McCoy 1981). The status of urban Appalachian children, however, apart from issues revolving around their education, remains largely unexplored. In this chapter, we focus on the health issues affecting Appalachian children living in the greater Cincinnati area. We delineate the health status of these children by comparing them with other children from metropolitan Cincinnati and with black children from families with a socioeconomic status similar to that of theirs.

The Cincinnati metropolitan area has an extensive history of Appalachian inmigration and an equally extensive collection of current social research comparing urban Appalachians with non-Appalachian whites and blacks. Although the data we use focus on Appalachian children in the Cincinnati area, we believe that our findings can be extrapolated to urban Appalachians living in other, similar metropolitan areas outside Appalachia.

PREVIOUS STUDIES

Studies conducted in Appalachia on the health of Appalachian children have concentrated primarily on mental health (Abbott 1989; Loof 1971), although health care delivery (Mabry 1989) and the effects of pollution (Osborne et al. 1990) have come under more recent scrutiny.

The literature on Appalachian children living in urban areas outside Appalachia is sparse; it is composed primarily of curriculum manuals (Stafford 1979; Urban Appalachian Council 1989) and school studies (Borman, Piazza, and Mueninghoff 1983; Borman and Spring 1984; Wagner 1977). Current research on the health status of urban Appalachians is equally meager (Friedl 1983; Obermiller and Oldendick 1989); it is almost nonexistent for Appalachian youths in urban settings (Lower Price Hill Task Force 1990; McCoy and Watkins 1980).

THE CURRENT STUDY

In order to gain insight on the health status of children living in urban Appalachian neighborhoods, we examined five years (July 1, 1985, through June 30, 1990) of inpatient admissions to Children's Hospital Medical Center (CHMC) in Cincinnati, the only hospital in the area to admit young children. The data set contains demographic information including the zip code of the patient's residence and the primary discharge diagnosis. The diagnoses are grouped according to the ninth revision of the International Classification of Disease (ICD-9).

We performed standardized morbidity ratio (SMR) analyses on these data. The SMR analysis is the ratio of the observed frequency of specific discharge diagnoses among the Appalachian children to an expected frequency based on some other population. We use two comparison populations in these analyses. First, we compare the frequencies of discharge diagnoses of children from predominantly white Appalachian zip codes with frequencies of the same diagnoses among children from the city of Cincinnati as a whole. We identify five Appalachian zip codes on the basis of prior research; these establish the residential concentration of Appalachians in certain Cincinnati neighborhoods (Fowler 1981; Fowler and Davies 1972; Maloney 1974a, 1985). Second, we contrast discharge diagnostic groups from the five heavily white Appalachian zip codes with those from five low-SES, predominantly black zip codes.

To avoid the bias created by including multiple admissions per patient in the data set, we conducted the analyses using only one randomly selected admission per patient per year of the study period.

FINDINGS

The SMR method of analysis contrasts the hospital discharge diagnoses of children living in predominantly white Appalachian zip codes with those of children living in the city of Cincinnati as a whole and of children in predominantly black zip codes. Demographic characteristics of these three study groups are presented in Table 7.1. The number of children age 0 to 4 and 5 to 11 living in the Appalachian zip codes is approximately 1 percent lower than in the citywide zip codes and 2 percent lower than in the black zip codes. The Appalachian zip codes are more racially homogeneous than the black zip codes; the Appalachian zip codes are 95 percent white, whereas the black zip codes are only 72 percent black. The ranges in median income for the Appalachian and the black zip codes do not overlap; the black zip codes are poorer than the Appalachian zip codes. The median income for the city of Cincinnati is within the range of the median incomes of the Appalachian zip codes.

Table 7.1
Demographic Characteristics of Children (<18 Years) Admitted to Children's Hospital Medical Center (July 1, 1985, through June 30, 1990) from Predominantly White Appalachian Zip Codes, City of Cincinnati, and Predominantly Black Zip Codes

Zip Codes	Total Population	% by Age in Years			% by Race		Range in Median Income[a]	
		0–4	5–11	12–17	White	Black		
Appalachian	59,318	8.7	10.9	8.5	94.5	4.8	18,268	(L)
							28,077	(U)
Cincinnati	852,421	7.8	9.8	8.6	79.8	19.3	25,375 [b]	
Black	61,119	10.6	12.5	9.6	27.2	72.2	8.007	(L)
							16,707	(U)

Source: CACI , 1985.
[a] L = Lower (bottom of range), U = Upper (top of range).
[b] Median household income for the city of Cincinnati.

Admission frequencies are presented in Table 7.2. A total of 1,843 children under age 18 from Appalachian neighborhoods were admitted to CHMC during the five-year study period; they account for a total of 2,514 admissions. From the city of Cincinnati, 16,838 children were admitted; 2,691 children were admitted from the predominantly black zip codes. The average number of admissions of children who were admitted at least once during the study period is comparable among the three study populations: this average ranges between 1.4 and 1.5. The average length of stay in the hospital varies by 1 day among the three populations: the average length of stay for Appalachian children is 4.2 days; for children citywide, 5.1 days; and for black children, 5.2 days.

Table 7.2
Admissions of Children (<18 Years) to Children's Hospital Medical Center (July 1, 1985, through June 30, 1990) from Predominantly White Appalachian Zip Codes, City of Cincinnati, and Predominantly Black Zip Codes

Zip Codes	Total No. Children Admitted	Total Admissions	No. Admissions Included in SMR Analyses[a]	Ages in Years [b]		
				0–4 (%)	5–11 (%)	12–17[c] (%)
Appalachian	1,843	2,514	2,112	1,482 (70)	416 (20)	214 (10)
Cincinnati	16,838	23,019	17,316	11,721 (68)	3,590 (21)	2,005 (12)
Black	2,691	3,929	3,253	2,299 (71)	606 (19)	348 (11)

[a] These SMR analyses are based on one randomly selected admission per child per year of the study period. Therefore, the same child may be included more than once in the SMR analyses.
[b] Ages of children are included in the SMR analyses.
[c] This age group is not included in this chapter.

We find comparable percentages of children from each of the study populations in the three age groups. Between 68 percent and 71 percent of the admissions are among the children age 0 to 4; 19 percent to 21 percent of the admissions are among the children age 5 to 11; and 10 percent to 12 percent of the admissions are among the children age 12 to 17 years old. Although Table 7.2 presents data pertaining to children under age 18, this chapter focuses on children below 12 years of age because children 12 and older may be treated at hospitals other than CHMC.

The significant results of the SMR analyses are presented in ascending order by ICD-9 code in Tables 7.3 through 7.7. There is no other significance to the order in which the ICD-9 disease classifications are listed.

Table 7.3 displays the significant results of the SMR analysis contrasting children age 0 to 4 in the Appalachian zip codes with children of the same age from the city of Cincinnati as a whole. The children living in the predominantly Appalachian zip codes are

Table 7.3
Disease-Specific Elevated SMRs (Lower Limit of 95% CI > 1) for Children Less Than 5 Years of Age Admitted to Children's Hospital Medical Center (July 1, 1985, through June 30, 1990) from Predominantly Appalachian Zip Codes Based on City of Cincinnati Rates

ICD-9 Disease Classifications	SMR	(95% CI)
Intestinal infectious diseases	1.42	(1.1, 1.7)
Other bacterial infections and HIV infection	1.61	(1.1, 2.2)
Poliomyelitis and other nonarthropod-borne	2.33	(1.8, 2.9)
Other diseases due to virus and chlamydia	1.87	(1.5, 2.2)
Inflammatory diseases of central nervous system	2.11	(1.5, 2.8)
Diseases of ear and mastoid process	2.10	(1.4, 2.9)
Acute respiratory infections	1.66	(1.4, 1.9)
Other diseases of upper respiratory tract	1.58	(1.1, 2.1)
Pneumonia and influenza	1.39	(1.1, 1.7)
Diseases of genitourinary system	2.42	(1.8, 3.1)
Symptoms	1.61	(1.4, 1.9)
Fractures	2.35	(1.6, 3.3)
Contusion with intact skin surface	5.94	(1.1, 14.6)

Note: These SMR analyses are based on one random admission per patient per year of study period.

discharged more frequently from the hospital with diseases classified as viral or bacterial infections of the gastrointestinal, nervous, and respiratory systems; diseases of the genitourinary system; symptoms; and injuries and poisonings. The viral and bacterial infections include viral and bacterial meningitis; intestinal infections including infectious colitis, enteritis, and gastroenteritis; acute respiratory infections; and croup. Urinary tract infections are the most common disease of the genitourinary system. The "symptoms" classification includes convulsions, fever, unspecified respiratory abnormalities, and failure to thrive. The principal injuries are skull and thigh fractures and bruises. The frequencies of these specific discharge diagnoses range from 40 percent higher to almost six times the citywide rate for this age group.

Table 7.4 presents the significant results of the SMR analysis contrasting children age 5 to 11 in the Appalachian zip codes with those in all Cincinnati zip codes. The children from the Appalachian zip codes are discharged more frequently with viral and bacterial infections, diseases of the respiratory and genitourinary system, and injuries. The bacterial and viral infections are primarily strep throat, chicken pox with complications, and herpes infections. Ear infections and perforation of tympanic membrane account for the diseases of the ear. The most frequently diagnosed diseases of the genitourinary system are infections of the kidneys and urinary tract. The "superficial injury" classification includes primarily abrasions of the head and neck and insect bites. These classifications are similar to those in the findings presented for the children less than 5 years old in Table 7.3, but the SMRs are larger: these increased frequencies range from twice to almost 12 times the city rate.

Table 7.4
Disease-Specific Elevated SMRs (Lower Limit of 95% CI > 1) for Children 5-11 Years of Age Admitted to Children's Hospital Medical Center (July 1, 1985, through June 30, 1990) from Predominantly Appalachian Zip Codes Based on City of Cincinnati Rates

ICD-9 Disease Classifications	SMR	(95% CI)
Other bacterial infections and HIV infection	2.56	(1.1, 4.6)
Viral diseases accompanied by exanthem	3.70	(1.2, 7.7)
Other diseases due to virus and chlamydia	2.17	(1.1, 3.6)
Diseases of ear and mastoid process	4.11	(2.9, 5.6)
Diseases of genitourinary system˙	2.24	(1.4, 3.3)
Open wound of head, neck, upper and lower limbs	2.42	(1.1, 4.3)
Superficial injury	11.85	(4.3, 23.2)
Complications of surgical and medical care, not elsewhere specified	2.62	(1.5, 4.0)

Note: These SMR analyses are based on one random admission per patient per year of study period.

In none of the SMR analyses contrasting children from the Appalachian zip codes with children from the city of Cincinnati are the discharge frequencies for the Appalachian children significantly less than the expected frequencies based on children from the city as a whole.

Table 7.5 presents the significant elevated results of the SMR analyses contrasting children age 0 to 4 and 5 to 11 from predominantly Appalachian zip codes with children in the same age groups from predominantly black zip codes. Children less than 5 years old are discharged more frequently with diagnoses of viral diseases of the central nervous system, such as viral meningitis, and diseases of the genitourinary system, such as urinary tract infections. These two disease classifications are similarly elevated in the SMR analysis based on children age 0 to 4 living in all Cincinnati zip codes.

Among the children age 5 to 11, the Appalachian children are discharged more frequently with bacterial infections; diseases of the ear, digestive system, and genitourinary system; and injuries. With a few

Table 7.5

Disease-Specific Elevated SMRs (Lower Limit of 95% CI > 1) for Children Less Than 12 Years of Age Admitted to Children's Hospital Medical Center (July 1, 1985, through June 30, 1990) from Predominantly Appalachian Zip Codes, Based on Rates for Predominantly Black Cincinnati Zip Codes

ICD-9 Disease Classifications	SMR	(95% CI)
Children Less Than 5 Years of Age		
Poliomyelitis and other nonarthropod-borne viral diseases of central nervous system	1.40	(1.1, 1.7)
Diseases of genitourinary system	2.24	(1.4, 3.3)
Children Ages 5–11		
Other bacterial infections and HIV infection	3.15	(1.3, 5.7)
Diseases of ear and mastoid process	4.13	(2.9, 5.6)
Diseases of digestive system	2.56	(1.4, 4.1)
Diseases of genitourinary system	3.37	(2.1, 5.0)
Superficial injury	7.08	(2.5, 13.9)
Complications of surgical and medical care	2.87	(1.7, 4.4)

Note: These SMR analyses are based on one random admission per patient per year of study period.

exceptions, the elevated SMRs are comparable with the SMRs reported in Table 7.4, contrasting children age 5 to 11 from Appalachian zip codes with those from the city as a whole. The Appalachian children are discharged seven times more frequently than the children from the black zip codes with diagnoses of superficial injury. The frequency of diseases of the digestive system is almost three times as high among the children from the Appalachian zip codes as among the children from the black zip codes. This disease category includes such diagnoses as gastritis and appendicitis.

In the SMR analyses contrasting children from the Appalachian zip codes with children from the predominantly black zip codes, children from the Appalachian zip codes are discharged significantly less often with certain disease classifications than children from the predominantly black zip codes. (These lower SMRs are presented in Table 7.6 for children age 0 to 4 and in Table 7.7 for children age 5 to 11.) Children less than 5 years old living in the predominantly Appalachian zip codes are discharged less frequently with diseases of the respiratory system, diseases of the skin and subcutaneous tissue, congenital anomalies, symptoms, and injuries and poisonings. The respiratory diseases include pneumonia and influenza; the skin diseases include inflammations of connective tissue as well as skin infections and irritations.

Table 7.6
Disease-Specific Depressed SMRs (Upper Limit of 95% CI < 1) for Children Less Than 5 Years of Age Admitted to Children's Hospital Medical Center (July 1, 1985, through June 30, 1990) from Predominantly Appalachian Zip Codes, Based on Rates for Predominantly Black Cincinnati Zip Codes

ICD-9 Disease Classifications	SMR	(95% CI)
Pneumonia and influenza	0.68	(0.54, 0.85)
Chronic obstructive pulmonary disease and allied conditions	0.49	(0.41, 0.58)
Pneumoconioses and other lung diseases due to external agents	0.31	(0.03, 0.90)
Other diseases of respiratory system	0.63	(0.37, 0.96)
Diseases of skin and subcutaneous tissue	0.61	(0.38, 0.91)
Congenital anomalies	0.63	(0.43, 0.87)
Symptoms	0.82	(0.71, 0.94)
Intracranial injury, excluding skull fracture	0.60	(0.39, 0.84)
Open wound of head, neck, upper and lower limbs	0.44	(0.16, 0.87)
Poisoning by drugs, medicinal and biologic substances	0.54	(0.32, 0.82)
Toxic effects of substances chiefly nonmedicinal as to source	0.36	(0.20, 0.66)
Other and unspecified effects of external causes	0.30	(0.08, 0.66)
Supplementary classification of factors influencing health status and contact with health services	0.46	(0.18, 0.87)

Note: These SMR analyses are based on one random admission per patient per year of study period.

Table 7.7
Disease-Specific Depressed SMRs (Upper Limit of 95% CI < 1) for Children 5–11 Years of Age Admitted to Children's Hospital Medical Center (July 1, 1985, through June 30, 1990) from Predominantly Appalachian Zip Codes, Based on Rates for Predominantly Black Cincinnati Zip Codes.

ICD-9 Disease Classifications	SMR	(95% CI)
Other diseases of central nervous system	0.30	(0.03, 0.85)
Chronic obstructive pulmonary disease and allied conditions	0.30	(0.23, 0.38)
Other diseases of respiratory system	0.30	(0.03, 0.85)
Diseases of skin and subcutaneous tissue	0.56	(0.30, 0.96)
Symptoms	0.64	(0.42, 0.91)
Poisoning by drugs, medicinal, and biologic substances	0.45	(0.14, 0.94)
Toxic effects of substances chiefly nonmedicinal as to source	0.17	(0.00, 0.66)

Note: These SMR analyses are based on one random admission per patient per year of study period.

Children age 5 to 11 living in the predominantly Appalachian zip codes are discharged less frequently than black children with diseases of the central nervous and respiratory systems, diseases of the skin and subcutaneous tissue, symptoms, and injuries and poisonings.

DISCUSSION

The SMR analyses presented here are based on five years of inpatient admissions to the Children's Hospital Medical Center in Cincinnati, the only hospital in the area to admit children under age 8. Rates of admissions to other city hospitals increase with age; therefore, our analyses focusing on children less than 5 years old are based on a complete enumeration of all hospital admissions in this age group. The analyses focusing on children age 5 to 11 are based on a less complete enumeration of hospital admissions.

To assess whether admission rates to the CHMC differ among the three study populations by age group, we review the data presented in Tables 7.1 and 7.2. The data presented in Table 7.1 demonstrate that the percentages of children age 0 to 4 and 5 to 11 in the Appalachian zip codes fall between the percentages for the citywide and the predominantly black zip codes. The data presented in Table 7.2 show that for the same age groups the percentages of children admitted to CHMC from the Appalachian zip codes fall between the percentages for the citywide and the predominantly black zip codes. On the basis of these aggregated data, it appears that the admission frequencies do not differ by age group among these three populations.

The results of a standardized morbidity ratio analysis are partially a function of the population on which the expected frequencies are calculated. We selected the city of Cincinnati as the de facto public health standard. The children from the predominantly Appalachian zip codes in both age groups are hospitalized more frequently than children from the city as a whole for diseases classified as infectious and parasitic diseases, diseases of the ear and mastoid process, diseases of the genitourinary system, and injuries. These children are never admitted less frequently than their Cincinnati counterparts for any disease classification.

In the 0- to 4-year-old age group, the SMRs are less than 3, with one exception: contusion with intact skin surface. These SMRs are significant but low. The significantly elevated SMRs, however, are consistent among related diagnostic groups: infections and parasitic diseases, diseases of the central nervous system and sense organs, and diseases of the respiratory system. These results do not appear to be the statistical artifacts of multiple comparisons. Rather, the interrelatedness of the disease classifications suggests that the results are substantive findings.

The SMRs calculated for the 5- to 11-year-old age group are larger than those for the younger group. The Appalachian children appear to be diagnosed in fewer different ICD-9 disease classifications than their siblings aged 0 to 4 but suffer more frequent health problems than children of the same age group from the city as a whole. In view of the previous discussion in this section concerning percentages of children and admission frequencies by age group in the study populations, it appears that this age-related increase in the magnitude of the SMRs is not an artifact of admission frequencies to other hospitals, which differ between these two populations, but a real change in relative health with age.

To control for differences in socioeconomic status, we also selected zip codes containing predominantly poor, black residents to compare with residents in the Appalachian zip codes. The black children in both age groups are hospitalized more frequently than their Appalachian counterparts with diagnoses classified as diseases of the respiratory system, diseases of the skin and subcutaneous tissue, symptoms, and injuries and poisonings. The children from the black zip codes come from homes with lower median incomes than those from the Appalachian zip codes. The relatively high frequencies of hospital admissions and the low socioeconomic status observed among the children from the predominantly black zip codes are consistent with the often-observed positive correlation between low income and poor health status.

Among Appalachian children, however, higher incomes do not translate directly into better health status. Appalachian children are admitted more frequently for diagnoses classified as diseases of the ear and mastoid process, diseases of the genitourinary system, and superficial injury. These results are remarkable in light of the poor health status of the black children with whom the Appalachian children are being compared.

The fact that higher income does not always correlate positively with better health status for Appalachian children is consistent with the general principle that the key indicators of socioeconomic status include educational attainment and occupational status as well as income. Longitudinal research in Cincinnati has shown that the median income of urban Appalachians is similar to that of non-Appalachian whites, whereas Appalachian educational attainment and occupational status more closely resemble those of non-Appalachian blacks (Obermiller and Maloney 1991).

The selection of race as a surrogate measure of socioeconomic status introduces race as a potential confounder in the analysis. Therefore, we must assess the extent to which race alone might determine access to medical care and/or utilization of medical services. As we pointed out in the beginning of this section, these aggregated data demonstrate no difference between these two populations in admission frequencies by age group. Comparable percentages of children in each age group live in the Appalachian and the black zip codes. Also, the admissions to CHMC reflect the same percentages by age group for these two populations. On the basis of population, there is no indication that race affects hospital admissions in this city.

In addition, aggregate data based on relatively large populations can mask trends among subpopulations. In analyzing citywide and aggregated zip code data, health issues facing residents of individual neighborhoods may be lost. The health risks faced by these subgroups can be different and even more critical than those affecting the larger population. For example, the children (age 0 to 4) in one low-income Appalachian neighborhood in Cincinnati are admitted more frequently for diseases classified as toxic effects of substances chiefly nonmedical as to source (SMR = 5.15) and for viral diseases accompanied by exanthem (SMR = 11.04) than children from other low-income Appalachian zip codes (Lower Price Hill Task Force 1990).

CONCLUSION

Several conclusions are apparent from the results of the SMR analyses presented here. Children from predominantly Appalachian zip codes and children from predominantly poor, black zip codes have numerous health problems that require hospitalization. The health status of urban Appalachian children differs markedly from that of poor black children and from that of the general pediatric population of Cincinnati. The health status of poor black children living in Cincinnati is generally worse than that of their Appalachian counterparts. This disparity between black and Appalachian children, however, highlights the severity of the health conditions for which Appalachian youths are admitted to the hospital more frequently than black children. Children living in predominantly Appalachian zip codes have distinctive health care needs that differ from those of children living in predominantly black zip codes and in the city at large.

These findings raise a number of significant public health questions. What patterns of utilization of primary care facilities prevail among

Appalachian and poor black children? Do the rates of hospitalization for specific disease classifications reflect a delay in obtaining health care, or do these hospitalizations reflect underlying health risks in these two populations? Would strategies to improve preventive health behaviors and increase utilization of primary medical care facilities be more effective than strategies to eliminate unsafe conditions in these children's physical environments? Do the aggregate data mask significant differences in health status within the Appalachian community? The results presented here demonstrate that answers to these questions are a compelling concern, not merely a matter of academic interest.

8

Concerning Contamination:
Attitudes on Environmental Issues
among Urban Minority Groups

Phillip J. Obermiller and Andrew Smith

As recently as 1989 it was possible to publish a history of the environmental movement without acknowledging the interrelations of race, class, and environmental quality (see McCormick 1989). This situation is changing rapidly, however. Churches (Commission for Racial Justice 1987), governmental agencies (Allen et al. 1992; Urban Environmental Conference 1985; U.S. Environmental Protection Agency 1992; U.S. General Accounting Office 1983), the legal system (Hayes 1992), advocacy groups (Bryant and Mohai 1990; Delgado 1986), and the popular media ("EPA Debates" 1992; "EPA Has a New Emphasis" 1992; Kanamine 1992; "Living with Pollution" 1991; "Minorities Exposed" 1992; Sloan 1992; R. Taylor 1984; Tyson 1991; Zwerdling 1973) are becoming more aware of the impact of environmental degradation on poor and minority groups.

Academic interest in the subject is also substantial. Some researchers have focused on the social and psychological outcomes of living in highly contaminated communities (Cutter 1981; Edelstein 1987); others have studied the implications of social class on environmental concern (McCaull 1976; Morrison 1986; Morrison and Dunlap 1986).

Robert F. Bullard, an applied sociologist, combines the variables of race, class, and community in all of his investigations. In the early 1980s Bullard began to document the practice of locating dirty industries, landfills, dumps, incinerators, and hazardous waste storage and disposal areas in or near poor black communities across the South (Bullard 1983, 1990a, 1990b, 1992; Bullard and Wright 1985, 1987a, 1987b). Studies involving rural Appalachian people and the environment are relatively scarce (Bagby 1990; Keesler 1991); the literature dealing with urban Appalachians and the environment is even smaller (Lower Price Hill Task Force 1990). The existing literature shows, however, that

Appalachian people both in the mountains and in the cities often live in communities affected by serious environmental degradation.

Although an increasing number of studies focus on the impact of pollution on minority communities, relatively few seek to elicit the opinion of minority and poor people about their environmental concerns. The few opinion surveys that have been conducted are outdated (a study conducted in 1965, during the height of the civil rights movement, found little concern among blacks for environmental hazards) or are limited by sample size (as small as 28), special populations (college students), or focus (use of social psychological variables) (D. Taylor 1989).

The Cincinnati metropolitan area provides an excellent opportunity for comparative research on minority opinions about environmental issues because its two largest minority groups are blacks and urban Appalachians. In greater Cincinnati the black population is a racial minority of relatively low socioeconomic status, the urban Appalachians are a minority ethnic group of medium socioeconomic status, and the non-Appalachian whites are a majority group of comparably high socioeconomic status (Obermiller and Philliber 1987; Philliber 1981b).

In view of these characteristics, it is reasonable to expect that the three groups will differ in their opinions about environmental issues and costs. Theories of stratification and resource mobilization would lend credence to the hypothesis that non-Appalachian whites would be more concerned than the other groups about environmental issues and more willing to bear the costs related to having a clean environment (McCarthy and Zald 1973). Urban Appalachians, with roots in a rural and mountainous region, could be expected to be concerned about environmental issues, but less willing to undertake the related expenses because of their blue-collar occupations and incomes (Whitson 1988). Finally, because of the historical effects of slavery and their comparably low socioeconomic status, blacks could be expected to have less concern about environmental issues and to be less willing to bear the costs of a clean environment (Cleaver 1969; Meeker, Woods, and Lucas 1973). In the remainder of this chapter, we examine the accuracy of these expectations.

THE DATA

In fall 1989 the Behavioral Sciences Laboratory at the University of Cincinnati conducted its semiannual Greater Cincinnati Survey (GCS), a random-digit-dialed telephone survey; the data presented here come from the Hamilton County, Ohio, portion of that survey. The 880 adults interviewed included 125 black non-Appalachians, 575 white non-Appalachians, and 160 white Appalachians. Black Appalachians were deleted from the data set because of their small numbers and to avoid confounding ethnicity with race.

This study uses a series of questions placed on the GCS by the Hamilton County Solid Waste Planning District Policy Committee and by the Cincinnati-based Urban Appalachian Council. We rejected questions related to environmental issues that could be affected by locational or similar biases. For example, some jurisdictions in the county provide curbside recycling, but others do not; therefore, certain questions about recycling were invalid for the purpose of this study. In keeping with the methodological suggestions of Van Liere and Dunlap (1980), we employed 35 questions that probe not only preferences but also willingness to bear the additional costs in taxes or fees associated with addressing environmental concerns.

Two limitations should be taken into consideration in reviewing the results of this study. First, the data understate the number of Appalachians by at least half because we deleted black Appalachians and included third and subsequent generations of Appalachians in the "non-Appalachian white" category. Second, the data were collected primarily for descriptive rather than explanatory purposes; thus the secondary analysis of such data is quite limited in its explanatory power. Even with these constraints, however, the data set is the most current and most complete source of information on minority attitudes toward environmental issues in Hamilton County.

THE RESULTS

Table 8.1 is a comparison of the relative socioeconomic status (SES) of each of the three groups. When the variables of educational attainment, occupational status, and household income are combined into an index, race is a key factor in the outcome. Non-Appalachian blacks are significantly underrepresented in the high-SES category and overrepresented in the low-SES category. Just over 81 percent of the non-Appalachian blacks are in the medium or low categories; this is the case for 73 percent of the white Appalachians and 63 percent of the white non-Appalachians.

White non-Appalachians generally are of higher socioeconomic status in Hamilton County, while non-Appalachian blacks are of lower status. The white Appalachians fall between these two groups.

Table 8.1
Socioeconomic Status of Non-Appalachian Whites, Appalachian Whites, and Non-Appalachian Blacks in Hamilton County, Ohio, 1989

	Non-Appalachian Whites		Appalachian Whites		Non-Appalachian Blacks	
High status	$N = 208$	36.5%	$N = 46$	26.6%	$N = 27$	18.6%
Medium status	$N = 194$	34.0%	$N = 59$	34.1%	$N = 56$	38.6%
Low status	$N = 168$	29.5%	$N = 68$	39.3%	$N = 62$	42.8%

$p < 0.001.$

Table 8.2 shows that when respondents were given the chance to establish priorities among seven specific social problems, each of the three groups gave "pollution and the environment" a relatively low standing. The non-Appalachian whites ranked it fifth, the blacks placed it sixth, and the Appalachians ranked it seventh.

Table 8.2
Identification of Important Social Problems by Non-Appalachian Whites, Appalachian Whites, and Non-Appalachian Blacks in Hamilton County, Ohio, 1989

	Non-Appalachian Whites		Appalachian Whites		Non-Appalachian Blacks	
Drug abuse	$N = 82$	37.1%	$N = 20$	25.6%	$N = 56$	43.2%
Poverty and homelessness	$N = 38$	17.2%	$N = 17$	21.9%	$N = 16$	12.0%
Quality of education	$N = 32$	14.4%	$N = 8$	10.3%	$N = 13$	9.7%
Crime	$N = 29$	13.0%	$N = 5$	6.6%	$N = 15$	11.4%
Condition of infrastructure	$N = 13$	6.0%	$N = 15$	19.0%	$N = 4$	3.2%
Unemployment	$N = 5$	2.1%	$N = 6$	7.8%	$N = 15$	11.9%
Pollution and environment	$N = 20$	9.0%	$N = 3$	3.6%	$N = 11$	8.4%
Other	$N = 3$	1.3%	$N = 4$	5.1%	$N = 2$	0.2%

$p < 0.001.$

Tables 8.3 and 8.4 provide a more detailed look at the three groups' responses to specific environmental concerns, issues, and costs. Table 8.3 shows that the groups agree on 23 separate items; Table 8.4 shows statistically significant disagreement among the groups on 12 items.

Table 8.3
Environmental Questions for Which No Significant Differences Were Found Among the Responses of Non-Appalachian Whites, Appalachian Whites, and Non-Appalachian Blacks in Hamilton County, Ohio, 1989

Concern about
    Acid rain
    Air pollution caused by auto emissions
    Water pollution caused by sewage
    Destruction of wetlands and wilderness areas in Hamilton County
    Destruction of the earth's ozone layer
    Disposal of hazardous wastes (chemicals, paint, or used oil)

Should we raise taxes or fees on garbage disposal to make the air and water cleaner, or are they okay now?

Should people like you pay for garbage collection through taxes, or should they pay through direct fees for the garbage collection services?

Would you and your household be willing to separate your newspapers, bottles, and cans from your other garbage each week so they can be recycled?

Would you favor or oppose a law in your community requiring the recycling of newspapers, bottles, and cans by households?

Would you favor or oppose fines for households in your community that do not participate in mandatory recycling programs?

Would you favor or oppose using tax money to provide cash incentives to encourage voluntary recycling?

Favor or oppose requiring deposits on
    Aluminum or steel beverage cans
    Other types of cans
    Plastic milk containers
    Glass jars and bottles
    Plastic containers other than milk containers
    Newspapers and magazines

Favor or oppose special fees for
    Disposing of used car batteries (fees)
    Disposing of used oil (fees)
    Disposing of grass clippings and leaves (fees)
    Cleaning up old dumps in the county that are environmental hazards (tax)
    Incinerating instead of burying garbage (tax)

Table 8.4
Environmental Questions for Which Significant Differences Were Found Among the Responses of Non-Appalachian Whites, Appalachian Whites, and Non-Appalachian Blacks in Hamilton County, Ohio, 1989

Concern about air or water pollution caused by the disposal of garbage (non-Appalachian whites and Appalachians less concerned than blacks, $p = 0.0054$)

Favor or oppose raising taxes or garbage collection fees to pay for the additional cost of recycling? (blacks and Appalachians less in favor than non-Appalachian whites, $p = 0.0001$)

Prefer garbage generated in Hamilton County be disposed of inside or outside the county? (blacks and Appalachians less in favor than non-Appalachian whites, $p = 0.0019$)

Acceptable to have within two miles of your home
  Landfill for burying garbage (blacks less in favor than Appalachians and non-Appalachian whites, $p = 0.0002$)
  Recycling plant (blacks and Appalachians less in favor than non-Appalachian whites, $p = 0.0006$)
  Yard waste composting plant (blacks less in favor than Appalachians and non-Appalachian whites, $p = 0.0011$)
  Garbage composting plant (blacks less in favor than Appalachians and non-Appalachian whites, $p = 0.0007$)

Favor or oppose special fees for disposing of
  Old tires (blacks and Appalachians less in favor than non-Appalachian whites, $p = 0.0002$)
  Household chemicals (blacks and Appalachians less in favor than non-Appalachian whites, $p = 0.0046$)

Favor or oppose options for solid waste disposal
  More landfills in county (blacks and Appalachians less in favor than non-Appalachian whites, $p = 0.0339$)
  Yard waste composting plant (blacks and Appalachians less in favor than non-Appalachian whites, $p = 0.0235$)
  Mandatory recycling (blacks and Appalachians less in favor than non-Appalachian whites, $p = 0.0409$)

DISCUSSION

In Hamilton County the Appalachians, the black non-Appalachians, and the non-Appalachian whites differ in cultural background and socioeconomic status. Nonetheless, we find clear similarities in the three groups' attitudes toward environmental issues. Although other social problems take precedence over environmental concerns, the groups show strong unanimity on specific matters; they expressed the same opinions on two thirds of the 35 environmental items investigated in this study.

Among the remaining one third of the items, in which we found strong diversity of opinion, blacks and Appalachians agreed on 75 percent ($N = 8$) of the items. This finding shows that on items on which opinions diverge, socioeconomic status is more important than race in determining attitudes toward environmental issues in the county.

For the nation as a whole, income, education, occupational status, and race correlate strongly with political activism centered on environmental issues (Mohai 1985). These variables, however, are not associated very strongly with concern for environmental matters in the general population (Mitchell 1979, 1980, 1984). Our findings in Hamilton County sustain the latter conclusion. Age, place of residence, levels of pollution, and family composition may have much stronger associations with concern for the environment (Buttel and Flinn 1978; Cutter 1981; L. Hamilton 1985).

CONCLUSION

Although poor and minority groups in Hamilton County may be affected disproportionately by environmental problems stemming from industrial and municipal pollution, they are similar to mainstream groups in their opinions about environmental issues and costs. If this is true of the general population, concern for the environment is a theme that unites people across class, racial, and ethnic divisions.

III

Social and Educational Issues

9

A Case for Naturalistic Assessment and Intervention in an Urban Appalachian Community

David Barnett, Anne Bauer, Barbara Baker,
Kristal E. Ehrhardt, and Stephanie Stollar

Young children in urban Appalachian communities, like many others, are at risk for school failure. Borman (1991) stated that a set of harsh realities supports the need for culturally appropriate ways to meet the needs of families in urban Appalachian communities: (1) Appalachians have a dropout rate of significant concern, similar to that of other cultural groups often targeted for intervention; and (2) Appalachians in inner-city neighborhoods live in the poorest housing yet are often slow to take advantage of health and prevention services. In addition, children from low-income urban Appalachian neighborhoods have higher rates of identifiable learning problems than children from the city at large.

The effectiveness of early intervention in preventing school failure is widely acknowledged. In order to be successful, however, such services must be accessed by the community. In this chapter, we make a case for naturalistic assessment and interventions in working with families to support their children's education and development. In making our argument, we begin by reviewing the stereotypes and realities of being Appalachian and growing up in the inner city that affect early intervention services. We then describe assessment and intervention strategies that strive for ethnic validity—strategies grounded in an ecobehavioral model. In conclusion, we address the likelihood that this style of service delivery will fit the strong personal, kinship-based orientation of urban Appalachian neighborhoods and make recommendations regarding the implementation of this model.

STEREOTYPES AND REALITIES

Polansky and associates (1972) described Appalachian cultural themes that have emerged as negative stereotypes: dependency, fatalism, and the apathy-futility syndrome. These stereotypes may be grounded in the frustration of service providers who use traditional formats in gaining access and making changes in Appalachian communities. In recent years, these stereotypes have been replaced by efforts at understanding the diversity in Appalachian cultures. Meaningful variations have been found in language and interaction styles, kinship ties, and self-reliance.

Language and Interactional Styles

Heath (1983), in contrasting the interactional patterns of two Appalachian communities, suggested that the ways in which children learn to use language depend partially on the ways in which families are structured in the community, beliefs about possible roles that community members could assume, and the concepts of childhood that guide children's socialization. This variation in language use, unique to each community, supports Keefe's (1988b) argument for variations within Appalachian culture.

In regard to communication, Plaut (1988) stated that in Appalachian cultures needed information is gathered in the context of broader relationships. In other words, there may be a need to chat for a while before getting down to business. Starting with issues may invite ineffectiveness; in the Appalachian ethic of equality, which implies more horizontal than hierarchical relationships, cordiality typically precedes information sharing.

As for the issue of neutrality (the desire to appear similar to community), interactions may be directive as in many other ethnic groups but must not be coercive in helping the client to find alternatives (Tripp-Reimer and Friedl 1977). Sensitive topics are best approached with indirect questions and suggestions; individuals may be very sensitive to hints of criticism.

Kinship Patterns

Among Appalachians the parenting unit is made up of many households rather than of the nuclear family and forms a family group (Keefe 1988b). This family group provides mutual aid as well as emotional and moral support; it may emerge as the decision-making unit and the agent of social control regarding behavior. In urban Appalachian communities, geographic proximity maintains the continuity and strength of the kin group, whether the kinship ties are biological or fictive.

Dunst, Trivette, and Cross (1988) suggested that the Appalachian family is part of an informal social support network that mediates well-being and coping. The strong ties of this family group, they argued, provide tentative evidence explaining why Appalachians seek professional help for problems less frequently than non-Appalachians. The personal and social networks of distressed individuals are sufficient to buffer and alleviate most of the day-to-day stresses that occur in the urban Appalachian community.

Dunst and his associates suggested, however, that the birth and rearing of a child who differs from his or her peers is a less frequent occurrence in the native rural community, and consequently, network members are less likely to be able to offer advice or provide support that alleviates emotional distress. According to Dunst and his associates, Appalachian families in urban settings reported that the formal social support networks, particularly social services, public health, and mental health, were less helpful than Appalachian families. These Appalachian families, however, did not report that informal support networks were more helpful than non-Appalachian families.

Borman, Mueninghoff, and Piazza (1989) reported that Appalachian women, like those in other cultures, demonstrate an identification with place, a significant role in the family as providers of emotional strength, and a capacity to perform social liaison work to link the family with the larger community. In their "bowing to no one," they give their children a mixed message about the value of school success via conformity to school norms.

Additionally, Borman (1991) reported that children in urban Appalachian communities grow up in a context of special familial ties. Those social services that they use are located in their enclaved neighborhoods and are staffed by community members; in contrast, the school organization is bureaucratic and frequently is centralized and hierarchically organized rather than community based. In her interviews with youths, Borman found the sense of neighborhood to be a supportive, sometimes overly protective network of family and near-kin.

The Paradox of Self-reliance and Help Seeking

Because of their economic and social experiences, some Appalachians may have a profound sense of powerlessness (Beaver 1988). This perception, together with the patronizing and culture-dominating approach of the mainstream society (including service agencies), contributes to a lack of openness to helping professionals from the mainstream culture.

Keefe (1988c) suggested that Appalachian culture is marked by egalitarianism and a concern for "neighborliness" and exchange. Thus, Appalachians tend to perceive institutions and social agencies with fear and suspicion, having learned to approach with caution those who say they have come to help. Three characteristics of Appalachian culture contribute to the likelihood that Appalachian individuals seek informal rather than formal help: (1) an egalitarian ethic, including a dislike of authorities and institutions that set out to control behavior; (2) individualism, in which self-reliant behavior is idealized; and (3) personalism, whereby individuals are admired and judged on the basis of their personal achievements and qualities. A "personal" approach by a physician was demonstrated by Friedl (1983) to be the most highly valued factor in the quality of health care.

Borman, Piazza, and Mueninghoff (1983) reported that urban Appalachians expressed the persistent Appalachian values of independence and individuality in their child-rearing goals along with urban working-class values of obedience to authority and the desire to maintain an aura of respectability. Urban Appalachian parents reported apparently conflicting aspirations; although they did not value studiousness, they hoped their children would complete high school. These parents evidently believed that active engagement with life was more important than personal sacrifice in pursuit of a professional career. Nonetheless, they still desired that their children succeed in school.

These three general groups of characteristics, as related to communication and interaction styles, kinship patterns, and self-reliance, are inconsistent with traditional majority-culture strategies for early intervention. Traditional early assessment (multifactored assessment) and intervention strategies would be perceived as intrusive in many urban Appalachian communities. In addition, the traditional model has many limitations (Barnett, Macmann, and Carey, 1992).

For example, assessment strategies may be unrelated to the reason for referral and may emphasize "within-child" characteristics that lead to deficit-based interventions. This traditional model typically has led to labeling and placement in special education rather than to mutually established goals and effective interventions. An alternative assessment and intervention model is needed to provide appropriate services to urban Appalachian communities. We propose naturalistic assessment and intervention strategies to meet that need.

NATURALISTIC INQUIRY

Many people may view professional practices associated with intervention design as discordant with naturalistic inquiry. Significant points of agreement and actual convergence may exist, however. We use the analysis by Lincoln and Guba (1985) in examining key issues to assert naturalistic principles for professional practice.

The Nature of Reality

The meaning of behavior is constructed in the context or setting. Multiple viewpoints usually need to be evaluated both holistically and in detail. Impressions of reality are likely to diverge considerably and must be taken into account. Whereas prediction and control are viewed as unlikely on the basis of naturalistic inquiry, these are not necessarily the same as professional practice goals, as we will discuss later.

The Relationship of the Consultant to Others and to the Problem Situation

Consultants (a term used to describe outside agents with technical expertise and the goal to help with the problem-solving process) necessarily are subjective in their approach to problem solving (Barnett 1988). Furthermore, they interact with individuals and problem situations.

Generalizability

"The aim of inquiry is to develop an idiographic body of knowledge in the form of 'working hypotheses' that describe the individual case" (Lincoln and Guba 1985, p. 38). With regard to intervention design, replications are used to study generalizability.

Causality

Lincoln and Guba (1985) state: "All entities are in a state of mutual simultaneous shaping so that it is impossible to distinguish causes from effects" (p. 38). This also is a foundation of assessment for intervention design. The unit of analysis is the mutual influence of behavior, person variables, and environment (Bandura 1986). Furthermore, it is assumed that complex behavior has multiple determinants. Functional assessments are used to describe meaningful units of behavior for which control is possible and desirable (e.g., school-related skills, harmful behavior).

The Role of Values

"Inquiry is value-bound" (Lincoln and Guba, 1985, p. 38) in several ways: (1) by values that are used to define problems and policy; and (2) by theory or paradigms used for problem solving (Bandura 1969). "Inquiry is either value-resonant (reinforcing or congruent) or value-dissonant (conflicting). Problem, evaluand, or policy option, paradigm, theory, and context must exhibit congruence (value-resonance) if the inquiry is to produce meaningful results" (Lincoln and Guba 1985, p. 38).

NATURALISTIC ASSESSMENT AND INTERVENTION GOALS

On the basis of research in education and developmental psychopathology, early intervention has been found to be vital for children who present severe instructional or parenting difficulties and for children who have minimal positive experiences with peers. The children may be described as hard to parent, teach, or befriend. The descriptive terms shift the emphasis from the child's characteristics to problem situations embedded in the family, the community, and the classroom. Some of these children may be characterized more traditionally as "disabled," but many others are not. The identification of these children is guided by the need to restore or improve the functioning of groups (family, classroom, peer) for the well-being of all group members. Thus, analysis focuses on natural systems such as families and schools, on mutually established goals, and on the roles and contributions of caregivers and peers who have the greatest opportunity to interact with the child experiencing difficulties.

When guided by intervention design, the key tasks for assessment relate to (1) defining problem situations, (2) determining goals and strategies for changing behaviors, and (3) evaluating not only environments in which to support change but also the possible roles of caregivers, family members, and peers. The nature of assessment for intervention design requires ongoing problem solving rather than fixed "answers" to a set of "given" questions (Schon 1983). The steps are guided by a consensus on the overall reasonableness of actions that depend on the problem situation. Thus, in contrast to decisions based on diagnosis or classification, the development of ecologically based helping strategies involves sequential decisions. Selection of target behavior and intervention involves a progressive process whereby plans are developed, implemented, maintained, evaluated, and modified as necessary.

NATURALISTIC INTERVENTION STRATEGIES

Naturalistic strategies emphasize that assessment and intervention must occur in significant settings and with caregivers who have the greatest opportunity to interact with the child. Fawcett, Mathews, and Fletcher (1980) argued that contextually appropriate interventions are more likely to be adopted. On the basis of their analysis, desirable interventions are: (1) effective, (2) inexpensive, (3) decentralized (i.e., controlled by local groups), (4) flexible enough to permit input by participants, (5) sustainable with local resources, (6) simple or comprehensible, and (7) compatible with the perceived needs, values, and customs of the setting.

Ethnic Validity

Ethnic validity may be defined as "the degree to which the problem solving process is acceptable and viable for the client in terms of characteristics associated with that individual's ethnic/cultural group and individual life experiences" (Barnett et al. 1991). In order to address the individual needs of urban Appalachian children and families, one can take several steps toward achieving ethnically valid practices. Barnett, Macmann, and Carey (1992) suggest that

these steps are not related to a search for "unbiased" developmental measures. In contrast, they include: 1) establishing an advocacy role; 2) understanding and accepting cultural differences related to the population being served; 3) involving professionals and other community members of the same cultural/ethnic/linguistic background in the problem solving and decision process to help "anchor" the cultural appropriateness of assessments and interventions (Savage and Adair 1980); and 4) using consultative and behavioral approaches to intervention design. (pp. 21–43)

An ethnically valid approach (as noted above) assumes that assessment occurs in significant settings, with caregivers and peers who have the greatest opportunity to interact with the child and are most familiar with the child. This approach also is known as "naturalistic" in that it is grounded in the natural teaching styles of successful caregivers (e.g., Hart 1985).

Consultation and Mutual Problem Solving

Consultation between parent and teacher, a collaboration problem-solving process, serves as the framework for naturalistic assessment and intervention. This process, as delineated by Gutkin and Curtis (1982), involves the following steps:

1. Defining and clarifying the problem.
2. Assessing and diagnosing the problem.
3. Brainstorming interventions.
4. Evaluating and choosing among alternatives.
5. Specifying consultee's and consultant's responsibilities.
6. Implementing the chosen strategy.
7. Evaluating the effectiveness of the action and recycling if necessary.

The consultation model assumes that parents and teachers have "expert" knowledge of the child (i.e., Bailey 1987; Dunst and Trivette 1987; Gerber and Semmel 1984). Yet although participants have been given "expert status," they must remain open to revising personal hypotheses and changing plans on the basis of findings of the assessment and of outcomes of intervention. During the problem-solving process, two assessment techniques—interviews and observations—adequately address the needs of a naturalistic model. Through the use of these techniques, assessment questions are answered with information that leads directly to the plausibility, discovery, or enhancement of naturalistic intervention strategies.

Ecobehavioral Interviews

Interviews have two important functions: "scanning" problem behaviors and circumstances, and analyzing problem situations in depth (Peterson 1968). The "waking day" interview (Wahler and Cormier 1970) and the problem-solving interview (Alessi and Kaye 1983; Kanfer and Grimm 1977; Peterson 1968) perform these functions. The waking day interview may be used to map the relevant features and sequence of family events, rules, and expectations for behaviors and objectives. The problem-solving interview helps (1) to define problem behavior, (2) to set priorities among problems, (3) to estimate the severity and generality of problems, (4) to determine antecedents and consequences of behavior, (5) to establish expectations for improved behavior, and (6) to suggest intervention strategies to be attempted by caregivers.

Observations

Participants should conduct observations in the child's natural environment (e.g., home, school, or day care) at carefully selected times, in order to analyze specific skills and behaviors, to understand ecological and cultural influences, to examine meaningful antecedents and consequences of behaviors, and to evaluate effectiveness of interventions. Possible recording methods include real-time recording; time-sampling methods such as the Preschool Observation Form (POF) (Bramlett 1990) and the Antecedent-Behavior-Consequence Analysis (ABC Analysis) (Bijou, Peterson, and Ault 1968; Bijou et al. 1969); participant observation; and self-observation (Bornstein, Hamilton, and Bornstein 1986). Barnett and Carey (1992) recommend that real-time observations should be used initially to help to determine natural units of analysis, target behaviors, and situational antecedents and consequences. Next they suggest structured observations should be used in order to clarify the problem further and to determine specific qualities and dimensions of behaviors.

Naturalistic Intervention Design

The most significant elements of intervention design depend on the roles of responsive and capable adults and on safe environments that support a wide range of learning objectives including peers, interesting learning materials, and functional activities. Initial intervention efforts may be related to assisting adults who are available to children and who are capable of fulfilling these roles. Naturalistic principles in intervention design enhance acceptability and generalizability.

Naturalistic intervention design emphasizes caregivers' existing competencies and thus may strengthen the caregivers' self-efficacy.

Children who are hard to teach or parent may have devastating effects on caregivers' self-confidence.

These interviews and observations may reveal that caregivers use techniques that are consistent in at least some ways with other successful or empirically based interventions. Yet the caregivers may not be aware of the importance or the logical extensions of their behavior. Therefore, an important role of the consultant may be to evaluate the emerging skills of caregivers, which can be enhanced through consultation, practice, and feedback. Planning can be directed to caregivers' naturally occurring approximations to successful strategies.

Thus, naturalistic intervention design includes modifying or extending caregivers' interventions or identifying interventions that may be incorporated easily into their routines. Plans for naturalistic interventions are based on analysis of caregivers' actual roles, routines, skills, and interests (Barnett, Macmann, and Carey 1992). Assessment plans can be directed to the identification of (1) an array of treatment options based on research and functional analysis; (2) naturally occurring parents' or teachers' intervention strategies that are likely to succeed as implemented or to become successful with change, guidance, and feedback; or (3) interventions that may be adapted to evident styles of parenting or teaching.

In summary, interventions are selected on the basis of a combination of strategies, including the analysis of situations through collaborative problem solving as well as the consideration of research and naturalistic bases for interventions. The naturalistic basis is determined by caregivers' evident skills, emerging skills, and accessible skills. Of interest to the consultant are successful naturalistic strategies, partially successful strategies, and skills that may be built upon, as well as the interventions that may readily fit caregivers' roles, skills, and situations.

ASSESSMENT IN URBAN APPALACHIAN COMMUNITIES

Borman (1991) recommended that social service delivery systems that are ethnically appropriate for urban Appalachian communities should address people's needs in their neighborhoods so as to emphasize personal attention and practical applications. Through an emphasis on an analysis of parents' actual roles, routines, skills, and interests, and through the use of caregivers' existing competencies, naturalistic assessment and intervention appear to be ethnically valid for these communities.

Language and Interaction Patterns

Plaut (1988) discusses a kind of cordiality and interaction foreign to some professional rules of conduct in initiating information sharing. This discussion is one way in which naturalistic assessment is appropriate to urban Appalachian communities. The waking day interview, one of the basic assessment tools of naturalistic intervention, employs natural discourse through its use of narrative and contextual "storytelling." For example, rather than asking, "What are your child's behaviors that concern you most?" the professional using the waking day interview could say, "It's sometimes rough getting everybody going in the morning. What about getting up and getting to breakfast?" This question invites a personal description of behavior rather than a comment potentially critical of a family member. The use of apparently indirect questions may meet the cultural need for neutrality and may avoid value judgments on other people's behavior (Tripp-Reimer and Friedl 1977).

Tripp-Reimer and Friedl (1977) suggest that in regard to neutrality, the professional should be directive but not coercive in helping the client to find alternatives. The collaborative problem-solving approach, which develops through interviews and observations, uses the caregivers' emerging skills as a basis and (as mentioned earlier) enhances these skills through consultation, practice, and feedback.

Kinship Patterns

Keefe (1988a) recommended that because of kinship issues, consultants should consider the family rather than the individual as the basic unit of treatment. Support should be sought within the family (Keefe 1988b). Naturalistic assessment and intervention, rather than addressing the child's needs in isolation, emphasize the child's interactions within the family. This approach is based on the availability of a nurturing caregiver; in urban Appalachian communities, several such caregivers may emerge as intervenors with individual children.

Self-reliance

Naturalistic interventions respond to the need for recognition of self-reliance in that individuals indeed solve their own problems through collaborative problem solving. The successful aspects of the parents' interaction with their child are emphasized, and approximations of more productive interactions are shaped. The caregivers' personal achievements in interacting with the child are used as a basis for further intervention, in response to the personalism common in the culture.

SUMMARY

The use of naturalistic assessment and intervention strategies seems to be congruent with general characteristics in urban Appalachian communities that may serve as criteria for achieving ethnic validity. Though the strategies described here address language and interactional styles, kinship patterns, and identification with place, perhaps the greatest strength of the strategy in this community is its emphasis on the parent's acting as a capable change agent regarding his or her children's behavior. This recognition of the individual's strength may connect professionals with parents in ways that enhance early intervention services in urban Appalachian communities.

10

Urban Appalachians and Professional Intervention: A Model for Educators and Social Service Providers

Lonnie R. Helton, Edwin C. Barnes, and Kathryn M. Borman

Educators and social service professionals who aspire to reduce system barriers in working with ethnic groups must establish priorities for understanding cross-cultural dynamics and formation of social values. A number of cultural analysts and community practitioners have emphasized the importance of such awareness in providing educational programs, family support, and social services to urban Appalachian families. Later in this chapter we present a model for culturally sensitive intervention with urban Appalachian clients based on parents' perceptions of and interactions with public school special education programs as well as with educational and social service programs housed in a neighborhood social agency.

Before examining cross-cultural interactional patterns, we consider the vantage points and motives characteristically held by professional social service workers and their ethnic clients at the outset of the helping relationship. According to Kleinman (1984), clinicians and service providers must be able to assess the personal meanings or intensity of identifications that a specific cultural context holds for individual clients. In addition, these professional workers must anticipate conflicts that may arise from clients' cultural identifications. The social meaning of differences related to ethnicity inevitably has a significant effect on shaping opinions, speculations, and emotions (Chestang 1982). Interaction with groups that hold different values thus can be considered "a quest for value-free perspectives," providing a base for culturally sensitive interaction (Spradley and McCurdy 1984). Most important, counseling and related emotional support services should be conducted with specific ethnic groups in ways that are culturally acceptable to these groups and that strengthen group members' feelings of participation and power (Green 1982).

In summary, this chapter examines the effect of a series of interventions undertaken by the authors with urban Appalachians. These were structured systematically to include urban Appalachian ethnic values and cultural perspectives. The dynamics of culture-specific interactions between social service professionals and members of this population will be considered in settings where urban Appalachians are encountered (Campinha-Bacote 1991). These interactions occur in schools or classrooms, in social service agencies, in community centers, and in urban Appalachian homes.

URBAN APPALACHIANS: COUNSELING AND SOCIAL SERVICES

Professionals working with urban Appalachian clients must understand their distinctive cultural values and beliefs because these values and beliefs affect the success of any intervention strategy. The characteristic values of familism, individualism, traditionalism, and fatalism especially characterize Appalachians as a rather homogeneous cultural population (Jones 1975; Weller 1965). Dillard (1983), for example, asserts that many Appalachian clients often require counseling not only because of differences in values but also because of their relative economic deprivation, the result of their limited access to social, economic, and political opportunities. As one of the principal spokespersons for the urban Appalachian community, Michael Maloney (1981) has long articulated similar issues and challenges facing Appalachians who live in economically impacted midwestern urban areas. In such areas, exclusion from access to policy-making forums may lead to the dislocation of such families and to a disruption of their indigenous social networks. Plaut (1988) and Keefe (1988c) emphasize separately that mental health providers who work with Appalachians need training to help them understand their own ethnocentrism. Such training is aimed at enhancing their empathy toward and appreciation of Appalachian cultural traits.

URBAN APPALACHIANS AND THE SCHOOL

In school, urban Appalachian children frequently are misunderstood and ignored by teachers and administrators; most of these individuals fail to recognize and address the incongruencies between middle American and Appalachian cultural values. Such discrepancies include definitive differences in child-rearing strategies, differing attitudes about the benefits of formal education, and dissimilar views regarding the advantages of mainstream cultural assimilation. In their school- and neighborhood-based research in a low-income urban Appalachian neighborhood, Borman, Lippincott, and Matey (1978) highlighted the control and power conflicts between urban Appalachian child-rearing practices and public school policies. In her more recent neighborhood-based work, Starnes (1990) explored teachers' attitudes toward urban Appalachian families and discovered that teaching strategies and communication with families are influenced negatively by teachers' stereotypic attitudes toward Appalachian culture. Because urban Appalachian children often lack the support needed to develop traditional values of school learning, they are likely to become apathetic and estranged in the classroom; the result is frequent absenteeism and school leaving (Borman, Piazza, and Mueninghoff 1983).

Collaboration strategizing by teachers, counselors, and parents of urban Appalachian children enhances both family solidarity and children's efficacy in learning at school (Borman, Lippincott, and Matey 1978; Starnes 1990; Wagner 1977). For instance, parents need to take part in regularly scheduled conferences with teachers and school administrators. In small-group meetings, all parties can look carefully at the child's learning needs and/or problems. Urban Appalachian families with children enrolled in special education classes have expressed feelings of inclusion and acceptance during such collaborative sessions. They appreciated being asked to voice their opinions and preferences and felt that direct contact with school staff members helped them to understand their children's strengths and weaknesses more clearly.

ETHNOGRAPHIC RESEARCH METHODS

In order to further assess the involvement of urban Appalachian families with educational and community programs, we conducted two separate qualitative studies between 1988 and 1990. These studies also were designed to result in policy recommendations to school personnel, agency counselors, and social service professionals. The first project, a qualitative case study, examined the level of participation by parents of children with disabilities in special education and social service outreach programs. The second project, an ethnographic field study, explored parenting skills groups in a community service agency with a sizable urban Appalachian clientele. The researchers used a variety of qualitative data-gathering techniques including direct observation, participant observation, and structured interviews with both urban Appalachians and service providers.

By using qualitative or ethnographic data collection methods, we were able, as far as possible, to see situations through the participants' eyes. Moreover, a qualitative approach seemed particularly appropriate in both studies because of urban Appalachians' preference for personal relationships and because "outsiders" seeking to provide professional services had an imminent need to develop rapport. We observed family responses to rearing a child with disabilities in the urban Appalachian home and neighborhood. Similarly, we observed urban Appalachian families receiving social services and counseling at a community center in a variety of interactions with professionals; Barnes also conducted in-depth interviews concerning culturally sensitive approaches to serving an urban Appalachian population.

The first study emphasizes urban Appalachian parents' views on how professionals might serve them best in school and in social service agencies. The second study explores how social service professionals attempt to bridge the cultural gap by continually providing services in keeping with Appalachian cultural values. Particularly through participant observation, and in-depth structured interviews, we learned how urban Appalachian parents respond to professionals in agency- and school-based conferences, in parent groups, and in meetings with various social service providers at home.

PARENTING A CHILD WITH SPECIAL NEEDS: URBAN APPALACHIANS AND THE SCHOOLS

The qualitative case study involved 20 poor and working-class parents and caretakers from 12 families of 13 children with developmental disabilities, ages 3 to 11. These 12 families, which were composed of couples, single parents, and three-generation units, were selected from neighborhoods throughout greater Cincinnati and northern Kentucky. Helton identified children who were thought to be either first- or second-generation urban Appalachians by reviewing charts at the diagnostic center where the children had been evaluated and by asking interdisciplinary team members involved in these evaluations to point out children of possible Appalachian heritage. Helton then telephoned the selected families to verify their Appalachian heritage and to determine the family members' willingness to participate in the study.

Helton also gave attention to each child's sex, age, type and degree of disability, family social class, and family configuration in order to achieve diversity in the sample. The sample included both first-generation parents (those born in Appalachia) and second-generation parents (those with at least one parent from the region). Nine of the children had varying degrees of mental retardation; the other four had a combination of learning disabilities, severe speech delays, and hyperactivity. All of the children had been determined to be developmentally disabled after extensive assessment at a local interdisciplinary diagnostic center.

After conducting structured interviews, Helton selected as key informants four families, two having children with mild mental retardation and two having children with moderate retardation. Subsequently, he carried out extensive observations, participating in family dinners, outings, and other events in their homes for eight months. Three of these families also arranged for Helton to observe their involvement in special education conferences at school, as well as their participation in community social service and/or recreational programs.

These children were enrolled in special education classes with low teacher–student ratios (a teacher and a teacher's aide for every 8 to 10 students). Each child's capabilities and progress were outlined and monitored through a uniform individual education plan (IEP), as stipulated by federal special education mandates. That is, each child had a written plan developed jointly at the beginning of each school year by parents, teachers, and school administrators and cosigned by all parties. This plan is reevaluated periodically by all parties and is revised according to the child's accomplishment of specific behavioral objectives in accord with Public Law 94–142 (1975). The highlight of such planning is that the parents of each child are involved in structured, collaborative meetings with teachers and school support staff to monitor and clarify the child's educational progress.

Common Patterns in Parents' Perceptions and Interactions

Several themes ran through the urban Appalachian parents' responses regarding their children with developmental disabilities. First, they responded more openly to professionals' displays of unconditional acceptance of their child, despite the child's delays in cognitive development, learning ability, and social adaptive skills. (We will elaborate on this theme in the next section.) These families accepted the limitations of their children with disabilities and advocated making the best of their strong points. They expected teachers, social workers, and others to do the same. In addition, most of the parents and caretakers perceived their children as making progress in special education; they highly valued the smaller classrooms, which afforded closer contact with the teachers.

Some parents, however, also believed that some school staff members made false assumptions about their children's performance and behavior. For example, the grandmother of nine-year-old Anna said that Anna's teacher often did not allow her granddaughter to perform simple self-help tasks such as putting on her coat. This teacher also criticized Anna for causing conflict with other children by bringing her stuffed animal toys to school. The grandmother of an eight-year-old boy, Sam, felt that the teacher was giving her grandson too much difficult homework. This grandmother said that the teacher never called her to discuss how Sam was doing, so she felt that she was "in the dark" about his classroom performance. She had learned to expect regular phone calls from Sam's previous special education teacher, whom she described as "taking more of a personal interest" in the boy and the family. The parents of nine-year-old Alan said that their son was wrongfully identified as a troublemaker and "always got blamed for fighting," although other children were involved. The mother added, "They only call me when there's something wrong, never any other time." Alan's teachers "pick on him because of who we are and where we live." Other parents were disappointed because the schools had failed to maintain regular contact with them about the school's expectations and their children's progress.

Unconditional Acceptance of the Child with Disabilities

As mentioned previously, both single parents and couples in the urban Appalachian community anticipated a level of acceptance by professionals consistent with the family network's inclusion of the child with disabilities. That is, the parents expected these professionals to treat their children with as much respect and recognition for their abilities as they received from family members. The mother of a nine-year-old said that her son is "just a little boy growing up." The father of a kindergarten-aged boy said that he would be able to accept his son's ability level in accomplishing either academic or vocational tasks and hoped that the school would work with the family in monitoring the child's progress so that realistic employment plans for the boy might be developed later.

Moreover, urban Appalachian families tended to see their children with disabilities in a sphere of "normality," more or less conforming to daily household and family routines and adapting within the neighborhood and community. The father of a five-year-old said that he did not expect his son "to build a rocket to the moon" but emphasized his wish for the boy to be able to get along with others, be happy, and make a good living. A grandmother said that the family does not use the word "retarded" in their home because labeling was oppressive to her nine-year-old granddaughter. She becomes quite excited about the little things her granddaughter is able to do, such as setting the table or going to the toilet by herself. Sometimes, she said, teachers and school staff members underestimated her granddaughter's "common sense" because of her handicaps; therefore, they often were overly protective or ignored her efforts to do things for herself.

Similarly, the aunt of one of the children, who herself is handicapped with moderate mental retardation, went through school in special education classes and now works at a computer terminal in a large corporation. The school and the vocational program in her community had labeled her "merely trainable" until her mother had insisted that she be given a chance to demonstrate her skills. She was displaying these skills already at home and in daily living activities.

In summary, urban Appalachian parents generally emphasized their children's positive points and expected school personnel to do likewise. Despite some differences of opinion with teachers, these parents still valued contacts with the school.

Interaction between Urban Appalachian Families and School Staff

Urban Appalachian parents acknowledge the usefulness of opportunities to collaborate at regular intervals with teachers and other school staff members such as physical therapists and speech therapists so as to learn better how to enhance their children's motor and language skills at home. More than half of the 20 parents and caretakers interviewed said that professionals know best how to help children and how to provide the types of expertise and intervention necessary for their children's overall progress. In fact, the young mother of nine-year-old Alan stated that she and her husband had moved from southern Kentucky back to the urban neighborhood where her family once had lived just so that her son, who had cerebral palsy, would have access to a better education than that provided by the rural district they had left.

Both the parents and the members of the extended family affirmed that they were satisfied with the capacity of their child with disabilities to acquire knowledge and functional skills in the classroom, through field trips, or in individual remedial therapy. All of these parents and family members encouraged their children to do homework and to practice such subjects as spelling and arithmetic. The mother of nine-year-old Pete drilled her son repeatedly each evening before he was allowed to call his friends or play with a neighbor child. Family members expected these children to abide by behavioral guidelines for the classroom and to learn as much as possible without undue pressure from the teachers.

At least 12 urban Appalachian parents of youths with disabilities expressed disappointment because the schools failed to notify them regularly about expectations and their children's progress in the classroom. The mother of a nine-year-old boy with learning disabilities stated that she heard from the teachers only when her son was in behavioral trouble in the classroom or on the bus. She and her husband expressed their frustration about school meetings, which the mother generally attended alone; she wanted to help her son to perform better in school and would "go to school to meet with teachers at midnight" if she knew this would help him. When the boy broke his leg and required a homebound teacher for several weeks, she was finally able to talk with the teacher, to observe her work with the boy, and to ask a number of questions about his learning needs. Like some of the other mothers and fathers who were interviewed, this mother appreciated the chance to talk with school officials during the IEP meetings; yet she felt that her input into goal setting was limited or was not addressed fully.

Helton observed that three parents were largely silent and passive during IEP meetings. They generally did not share their views spontaneously and were asked fewer questions as the meetings progressed. (The longer these parents remained silent, the less likely they were to be asked questions by the team during the meeting.) Near the end of the meeting, parents were asked to share concerns or ask questions. Two of the three parents lacked an understanding of medical and other professional terminology; yet they would not admit their confusion until after the meeting. The father of a five-year-old boy did not even like the use of the term *professional,* stating that professionals are "just like everybody else—some good, some bad." (The professional's presentation style and openness sets the stage for his or her ability to communicate with urban Appalachian parents.)

One grandmother was helping her divorced son to rear his nine-year-old, a child with moderate mental retardation. She said that the school had not made contact with her about Joe's progress during the early part of the school year. Consequently, she had not called the special education teacher even though she had specific questions about the appropriateness of homework assignments and Joe's readiness for certain kinds of academic work. She said that she assumed the teacher was not committed to helping her grandson; otherwise, the teacher would have kept in touch with the family, as last year's teacher had done.

A middle-aged couple with two sons, both of whom had severe disabilities, were disappointed that neither the school nor any of the social service agencies called them except to discuss trouble. As a result, they seemed to have a negative attitude toward these professionals, which greatly impeded intervention and carried over from the school to other settings.

Our major argument is that urban educators and social service providers must be culturally sensitive to Appalachian perspectives on health and well-being. A direct, no-nonsense approach is conducive to establishing trust, rapport, and compliance. Schools and support agencies that focus on client-centered, value-oriented intervention will bring about optimal change in the client's situation. Finally, professionals serving urban Appalachians may be apprised of these individuals' predilection for collaboration rather than unilateral service delivery, as shown in our discussion in the next section.

Preferences regarding Social Service Delivery

Several of the 12 families were followed continuously by social caseworkers, public health nurses, and/or parent trainers and appeared to prefer a home-based approach to intervention. One young mother of two boys, ages five and three, preferred this method as both boys had been enrolled previously in home-based Head Start programs. The parents resisted long-term psychodynamically oriented counseling and structured behavior management involving token reinforcement; they simply did not keep appointments.

One home trainer from a child protection agency, along with a public health nurse, helped a mother to control her 5-year-old son's disruptive and aggressive behavior through informal modeling of control techniques and gentle reinforcement of parenting abilities. Moreover, the relationship on which any intervention was predicated was generally as important as what was done during each contact. A 28-year-old single mother said about her agency-assigned nurse, "We go way back; we're more like friends, me and her." Parents especially resented social workers and special educators who neglected to ask them what they considered to be the child's and family's needs before devising plans for "amelioration." Sometimes the parents felt that information about family problems or concerns was not shared among the professionals involved, or that such details were not communicated as the child moved from one special education or social service program to another. Consequently, these parents lost faith in the ability of the school system to personalize their children's education.

These 12 urban Appalachian families relied on their rather extensive informal support networks of extended family members, friends, and neighbors for ongoing emotional and periodic tangible support. Families frequently thought that social service and educational staff members failed to ask them about their ability to "cope" in their own way with the problems of the child with disabilities. In fact, most of the parents studied were interested in participating in a parent support group, if available, in order to obtain emotional support, to share ideas with other parents on rearing a child with special needs, and to exchange information about community resources. Two parents had attended parent groups within the school system and had found them extremely helpful. They had become dismayed, however, by the poor attendance of other parents, which they attributed to the time and place set for these meetings. Parents expressed a strong desire for more joint decision making and mutual planning of intervention for their child. They often spoke about needing a parent group or forum "closer to home," in the neighborhood.

In summary, urban Appalachian parents of children with disabilities preferred to continue involvement with social service programs that provided ongoing, personalized, informal methods of service delivery and that took the needs of the entire family into consideration. Community-based programs were more accessible; community centers, such as the one described in the next section, provided an array of much-needed services including day care, crisis intervention, and parent education groups.

UTILIZATION OF COMMUNITY SUPPORT SERVICES AND ADVOCACY

In the second research project, a qualitative study of a large social service agency in northern Kentucky serving urban Appalachian clients, two areas of client-staff interaction appeared to be most significant in facilitating the development of skills and capacities in urban Appalachians: (1) support group discussion and demonstration of parenting skills and (2) provision of practical problem-solving techniques with follow-up. These services were provided to urban Appalachian residents in low-income neighborhoods in keeping with the agency's objective of promoting clients' self-help and decision-making capabilities.

The primary data sources in this project were two professional staff members—a family therapist/mental health counselor and a social worker—who served as key informants and allowed active participant observation in a parenting support group and in individual advisory sessions with clients. From these informants' responses to unstructured interview questions and from observations of their interactions with urban Appalachian clients over 10 weeks, we identified four focal points: routines and responsibilities, nonobligatory services, problem solving with clients, and cultural behaviors observed in clients.

Social service workers approached their urban Appalachian clients with different interactive styles and ethnic backgrounds, although they maintained comparable philosophies about client advocacy. One social worker, Sue McDonald, was observed attempting to explain city housing laws to several families who had failed to make regular rent payments and to maintain their property. Earlier sessions with the family members had focused on money management and rights to due process. These sessions had shown positive results when the family arranged for an arbitration settlement and saved enough money to pay their bills. The clients' cultural disdain for "keeping a calendar," however, compromised their sense of responsibility for making timely payments. Resolution was possible only after fiscal obligations were adjusted to a "seasonal" timetable. The social worker's efforts toward achieving this resolution were enhanced by her sensitivity to the Appalachians' unique reasoning coupled with her willingness to patiently explain urban social customs and residents' responsibilities.

Sue McDonald said that her comprehensive efforts for some of her Appalachian clients included advocacy work with municipal officials and grocery shopping for household necessities on behalf of the homeless. In her frequent advocacy for the Appalachian residents in the city, this professional worker was extremely effective in reducing their confusion about public assistance applications and about Aid to Dependent Children (ADC) and Women, Infants, and Children (WIC) program entitlements. On her own time, in order to prevent conflicts or the loss of Appalachian residents' legal rights through cross-cultural misunderstandings, she joined Appalachian neighborhood forums to discuss housing regulations and school board issues. Sue was an activist on behalf of her clients; she regularly provided more than simple didactic information when problems could not be resolved. In an interview, she commented, "Sometimes I'll just stop and listen, perhaps give them a hug if I know them and they're comfortable with such contact—that kind of support." Sue constantly urged her Appalachian clients to be persistent in the face of cultural barriers around them and supported their acquisition of the skills required to confront bureaucratic structures. Although her ethnic ancestry was not Appalachian, she achieved a rapport that enabled her to model appropriate social behavior and to help her clients achieve more productive lifestyles.

Similarly, the family therapist in the agency perceived that her role as a counselor and parenting skills educator gave her "entrée with a special community of people." Gloria Fine attributed her success in addressing problems affecting entire Appalachian families to an emphasis on the potentiation and individuality of each member. She "maintain[ed] sensitivity to traditional Appalachian mores but stress[ed] that urban Appalachian families should set mutual goals." Collaborative strategizing with parents and with key service providers and teachers often resulted in problem-solving approaches or in actual solutions based on the therapist's experiences. When urban Appalachian parents were involved regularly as "problem-solving partners," they were likely to adopt new child-rearing practices. Gloria initiated opportunities for both input from clients and careful, collaborative demonstration of parenting skills after she realized that didactic instruction alienated most Appalachians. She regularly scheduled optional parenting support groups whose agendas included how to engage in child discipline and constructive arguments with children, how to recognize and solve sociocultural problems, how to manage work or school responsibilities, and how to create family solidarity. For much of the time in her parenting sessions, each participant and family member was allowed to voice his or her other concerns and experiences. This opportunity for expression in a supportive environment was unprecedented and galvanizing for many of the clients. Gloria's consistent and equitable feedback on parenting issues allowed group members to recognize their own problem-solving abilities as well as the importance of family-focused goals.

Gloria noted in three separate interviews that she attempted to challenge her clients individually to raise their own expectations of what might be achieved. As a reinforcement technique, she was careful to point out their incremental weekly progress to them, especially if stresses from other problems, usually social or financial, went unabated. As an Appalachian ethnic herself, Gloria used her understanding of Appalachian values and history to form a bridge to her clients who had migrated (as her parents had done) to the city. Traditional Appalachian cultural values such as individualism, self-reliance, modesty, and strong familial orientation are apparent among Gloria's clients; consequently, she has altered her interactive style to make it compatible with theirs.

Her most difficult task was to persuade urban Appalachian residents to resolve economic, social, and psychological problems as they occur and to seek out assistance rather than denying their needs or presuming that service providers and professionals would not understand their customs and perspectives.

CONCLUSION

Our separate studies of urban Appalachian families and the social service providers who serve them in the community affirm the need for parent- and family-focused, culturally sensitive intervention in both the school and the community. These research projects are significant for their assessment of the quality of services provided to urban Appalachian families through the schools and community agencies. The emphasis on understanding family attitudes and experiences and on professionals' approaches to working with urban Appalachian clients helps to explain how social service providers can make their intervention plans more culturally sensitive.

In both the school and the community, urban Appalachian parents expected and responded best to personalized intervention methods grounded in respect for the individuality of each family member. Parents often found it difficult to manage their children's acting-out behaviors at home but were receptive to concrete, pragmatic demonstrations of effective disciplinary techniques. Parents also were interested in receiving practical, direct, clearly stated information to assist them in problem solving in connection with such issues as money management, finding housing, or applying for social services. Urban Appalachian families appreciated and gravitated toward school or agency profession- als who maintained open communication with them and showed enough concern to engage them in mutual goal setting.

These families also placed a high value on the quality of the education provided for their children with special needs; they seemed to trust the special education teachers and support staff members to serve as brokers for other important services such as adaptive equipment, tutoring, or recreational programs. Most of these parents expressed a strong interest in joining parenting groups at school or at a location in their neighborhoods. Urban Appalachian parents wanted professionals to be more accepting of both their children and their families and valued them for their personal and informal approaches to and communication with parents. The professionals also were appreciated because they showed respect for the parents' understanding of the child and for the needs of the entire family, and because they were direct in their relationships with the parents. The teachers, administrators, and school support staff members who were regarded most highly were those who treated the children as individuals, just as they would treat any other children, regardless of their disabilities or problems.

For professionals serving urban Appalachians in a large social service agency, family stability is a priority. More effort is needed to strengthen Appalachian family units while empowering individual members to attain self-care and to set goals. Whenever possible, additional service providers, teachers, and counselors should join in collaborations to diagnose problems and formulate solutions. This is particularly true when the problems originate in schools and institutions that are designed to be structured and impersonal (Wagner 1977). Interactive guidance on family and child-rearing issues should include concrete demonstrations of concepts and skills. As urban Appalachians experience individual and family conflicts, resolution strategies must be established early and followed up consistently. Urban Appalachians will be better able to improve their quality of life if these interventions are carried out with discretionary knowledge and sensitivity.

A CONCEPTUAL MODEL FOR INTERVENTION WITH URBAN APPALACHIANS

In this concluding section, we present strategies for intervention and a conceptual model for integrating those strategies with the hope that teachers, social service providers, and other professional workers might benefit (See Figure 10.1). Our model consists of four components: (1) family members' individuality and empowerment; (2) regular, culturally sensitive intervention with families toward mutual goals; (3) enhancement of child behavior and child-rearing skills; and (4) collaborative strategizing among parents and professionals. This model should benefit professional workers in the social services and allied fields by introducing a culturally sensitive framework that respects Appalachian cultural values and places the family at the center of service delivery efforts.

Family Members' Individuality and Empowerment

Because urban Appalachian families value their individuality and personal freedom and because they often feel powerless and culturally disenfranchised, this model of intervention will provide them with

Figure 10.1
A Model for Professional Intervention in the Urban Appalachian Family

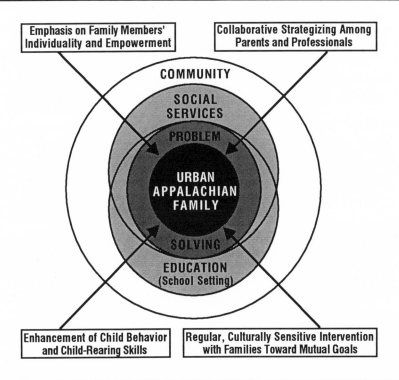

opportunities to feel included and respected during service delivery. A focus on individual behaviors and concerns in counseling and in the classroom can help both family members and professionals to develop a trusting relationship and can lead to greater use of services.

Regular, Culturally Sensitive Intervention with Families

Regular outreach services and ongoing communication with professional workers can create a more trusting environment for urban Appalachian families and service providers. These families often are threatened by, or uncomfortable with, the middle-class value systems of most professional workers; and frequently they feel that teachers and social service providers fail to include them in intervention plans for their children and themselves. The proposed model encourages parents and professionals to increase their capacity for setting mutual goals and expectations and to assess intervention plans for clarity and consensus.

Enhancement of Child Behavior and Child-Rearing Skills

Many urban Appalachian parents recognize a child's behavior problems at home or in school as well as acknowledge the need for the child to comply with regulations set by authority figures. Discussion of discipline and child-rearing practices at home and at school should be articulated clearly among all parties involved, and parents' "special knowledge" should be honored. Whenever possible, professionals should demonstrate effective parenting skills.

Collaborative Strategizing among Parents and Professionals

Mutual involvement and collaboration between family members and professionals will help families to feel more secure in the professional domain and to sense acceptance of their rights and responsibilities as a family. Through this approach, the Appalachian cultural values of personalism, individualism, and family solidarity will be respected and integrated carefully into service plans.

SUMMARY

A more culturally sensitive and individualized intervention approach to urban Appalachians is possible if the families' concerns and priorities are central to all forums for decision making and problem solving in schools and social service agencies. Educational and socially empowering intervention strategies can be implemented most effectively with urban Appalachian families through recognition of their cultural values, the integrity of parental involvement, and the individuality of each child. Children should be given didactic information and counseled on skills for practical living in a manner that instills cultural pride and also raises their own expectations for learning. Actual and perceived patterns of apathy in the urban Appalachian community will be diminished only through activism and coalitions among schools, social agencies, and families. As our intervention model shows clearly, the urban Appalachian family must be brought into focus as the central system for engagement in effective problem solving and attainment of goals in service delivery.

11

Echoes from the Hill: Urban Appalachian Youths and Educational Reform

Elizabeth M. Penn, Kathryn M. Borman, and Fred Hoeweler

I've seen a cultural turnover. Way back in the 1950s, the coal business went down on account of the oil. Coal was priced off the market, and after World War II, the coal miners of the mountains had to go somewhere, so they flocked to the cities. They jammed the inner city and blockbusted the inner city. When these mountain people started coming across the bridge into Cincinnati, people started selling their shops and places in Over-the-Rhine and moving out, and these people moved into these places. Along about the same time, you had the cotton picker and cotton setter. A lot of your tenant farmers had to go somewhere because machinery took over the cotton fields. At the same time, you had the blacks coming from the Delta. They were coming from the woods and everywhere, from Mississippi, Louisiana...landing here and wherever, mostly in Michigan. Michigan got the biggest batch of them, and Chicago. When they did [migrate], they brought along cultures with them. You can go down to Laurel Homes and you have your tub outside with a fire in it, screen over the top, doing your barbecuing in the evenings. You could smell barbecue all over town when they first got here.

Ernie Mynatt, 60-year-old social activist

During the 1940s, a booming war-stimulated economy in Chicago, Detroit, Cleveland, and Cincinnati drew hundreds of thousands of migrants from the Appalachian region. In the 1950s, the automation of coal mining and the development of alternative fuel sources drove tens of thousands from the Kentucky and West Virginia coalfields. Finally, during the 1960s, additional migrants streamed to the same cities. Wagner (1987) and others who have examined the effects of this massive movement from rural to urban places speculate that this huge demographic shift went largely unnoticed because these almost 3 million migrants were white *and* their migration took place *within* the United States.

The key protagonists of our research are 152 urban Appalachian youths who participated in the 1991 Summer Program. Their household sizes range from one person to nine; the modal household contains four family members. The average annual family income reported by these youths is $7,788. Per capita income varies; the highest average per capita income ($12,312) is reported by those living in two-person households. Program participants have aspirations far beyond their current circumstances, and they believe they are capable of achieving their goals. Unfortunately, their aspirations are not matched by their academic achievement. In this chapter, we explore urban Appalachian adolescents' academic achievement. The next section of this chapter examines the crisis in educational achievement facing urban Appalachian youths who live in enclaves. In the sections that follow this initial analysis, we repeat the words of the youths themselves as they describe their failures and the failures of the system. We hear them describe the need for "more personal" schooling, more cultural sensitivity in the face of multigroup social tensions, and more connections with their neighborhood and their community. Finally, we make specific recommendations to address each of their concerns.

ACADEMIC FAILURE

Urban Appalachian adolescents have the highest school dropout rate in Cincinnati proportionate to their numbers (Borman 1991). Urban Appalachian neighborhood enclaves in Cincinnati rank higher than either predominantly black or other white areas both in the percentage of high school dropouts and in the percentage of the population age 16 to 25 who are neither high school graduates nor currently attending high school. Even those students who remain enrolled in school are achieving at significantly lower levels than their non-Appalachian peers.

The young people from Cincinnati's Lower Price Hill recognize that the Cincinnati public school system is failing to meet their needs. Participants in the Summer Program eloquently articulate their perceptions of the educational problems experienced by urban Appalachian youths. They also make recommendations for decreasing the dropout rate, for improving the quality of their school experiences, and for raising the level of their academic achievement.

In 1974, Michael Maloney (1974a) predicted that the educational situation for these youths would not improve but would continue to deteriorate. Almost 20 years later, his contention is supported by data from the Summer Youth Program. The state of Ohio requires that all participants in the federally funded job skills program take the Wide Range Achievement Test (WRAT), Level II. WRAT scores are reported in grade-equivalent form. The grade norms were derived from the mean grade levels of the participants in the normative sample; the test's authors note, however, that these grade placement measures may not be precise (Egan 1977). Because of the limited number of items at any given level, the WRAT cannot establish students' specific strengths or weaknesses. It can, however, indicate the need for further assessment of a student's achievement. Even this limited assessment suggests that the Summer Program participants are functioning well below the levels of their non-Appalachian peers. The scores of the 152 program participants reveal a gap of one to three years between the students' actual grade level and their grade-equivalent scores on the WRAT. The gap is larger in verbal achievement than in mathematics; and the difference is greater for black participants than for white (see Table 11.1).

Table 11.1
Average Wide Range Achievement Test Grade-Equivalent Scores for 152 Summer Program Participants, 1991

	Total Population, $N = 151$	
Avg Gr Equiv	Avg Math Gr Equiv	Avg Verbal Gr Equiv
9.49	7.72	6.25
Difference	1.7	3.24
	White Participants, $N = 130$	
Avg Gr Equiv	Avg Math Gr Equiv	Avg Verbal Gr Equiv
9.52	7.80	6.22
Difference	1.72	3.30
	Black Participants, $N = 21$	
Avg Gr Equiv	Avg Math Gr Equiv	Avg Verbal Gr Equiv
9.7	7.0	6.28
Difference	2.7	3.42
	Male Participants, $N = 71$	
Avg Gr Equiv	Avg Math Gr Equiv	Avg Verbal Gr Equiv
9.46	7.75	6.24
Difference	1.71	3.22
	Female Participants, $N = 81$	
Avg Gr Equiv	Avg Math Gr Equiv	Avg Verbal Gr Equiv
9.51	7.69	6.25
Difference	1.82	3.26

The WRAT scores are consistent with data from the Lower Price Hill Task Force (1990), which show that children from low-income urban Appalachian neighborhoods have higher rates of identifiable learning problems than children from the city as a whole. In the Cincinnati Public Schools, achievement scores on the California Achievement Test (CAT) generally have declined for children in grades 1 through 6; during the past five years the decline for urban Appalachian children was two to three times greater than for the district as a whole (Lower Price Hill Task Force 1990). In view of the CAT results for children in these grades, it is not surprising that the adolescents' WRAT scores are also poor in relation to national norms. Clearly, the urban Appalachian youths encounter difficulty in schooling. Additional data are necessary to identify specific problems and solutions.

Even without access to the data described above, the adolescents are aware that they and the members of their neighborhood reference groups are not succeeding in traditional urban high schools. They express their perceptions and frustrations regarding their academic failures.

DESIRE FOR MORE PERSONAL ATTENTION

One student would like school to be more personal:

They seem to push you away and put you off. One of the boys said that there are a few teachers who will help you and become involved but not many. (Jay, 17-year-old student)

The need for more personal attention is expressed frequently by urban Appalachian students who were interviewed during their participation in the 1991 Summer Program. For some, "personal" translates into more individual attention in the classroom. In a group interview, one 16-year-old girl stated:

There should be less kids in a classroom. It would be better. Like when they're teaching something and you don't understand, and they just go on—not to just go on. The teacher knows a student does not understand when you give them stupid faces or raise your hand and tell them you don't understand. Or say, "Excuse me, teacher, I don't understand." You can tell....Body language can tell, or some may call on you....You know how Miss Adams—when you wouldn't understand what they was doing, when she called on you, you'd get part of it right, but then you don't know the rest and she'd say, "Well, try to figure it out."

Her peers agreed. One girl remarked, "They need some teachers that like to help and that, 'cause half the teachers that I got, they don't want to help the kids." The girls did not attribute the absence of personal attention entirely to the teachers. Some "classes are small, but they go to, like, thirty, thirty-five....In a lot of my classes this year we had to share books—like three and four of us—because they didn't have enough."

Only one dissenting voice was heard in this interview. Katie, who attends a small parochial girls' school, said: "At my school, they go over it again and again 'til you know it by heart. If you fail half of it, you go to a different teacher and they teach you all over again." Each of these students perceived advantages in a school social climate that includes small classes and individual attention from teachers. Their perceptions are supported by extensive research on effective schools (Meade 1991). Both Katie and Mitch, a student in an alternative program, chose to attend schools that they perceived to be "more personal." Katie's family can afford to pay parochial school tuition, and Mitch qualified for an alternative public high school program. Most of the adolescents interviewed, however, do not have such a choice; they attend a large public urban high school without a special curriculum.

Social climate is among the reasons cited frequently by poor urban parents who choose to make extreme financial sacrifices for private and/or parochial education for their children. Erickson (1981, p. 6) argues that "the desire for a more stable, constructive social climate, where learning is actively, consistently promoted, is a major part of the explanation" for parents who remove their children from large urban schools. The social climate includes less bureaucratic regulation, the potential for parental involvement and input, and a "reasonable homogeneity of viewpoint in the constituency."

Rutter (1979) draws similar conclusions from research on effective schools in Great Britain. He includes the following elements in his definition of social climate: "degree of academic emphasis, teacher actions in lessons, the availability of incentives and rewards, good conditions for pupils and the extent to which children are able to take responsibility" (p. 178). Rutter also suggests that the cumulative effects of these factors are greater than the effect of any single element. Those who have experienced the Appalachian culture suggest that these personal elements of social climate may be even more important for the Appalachian parent and child than for members of other American minority cultures.

In *Yesterday's People*, Jack Weller (1965) uses Herbert Gans's concept of "person orientation" to characterize Southern mountain society. Whereas the object-oriented individual may strive toward an external goal such as a college degree, the person-oriented individual desires

to be a person within the group. He wants to be liked, accepted, and noticed, and he will respond in kind to such attention. He is reluctant to separate himself from any group in which he finds this acceptance. His life goals are always achieved in relation to other persons and are a product of participation in the group. Without such a group, the goals cannot be achieved. (Weller 1965, p. 50)

Weller's characterization is not only supported by the statements of the students in the Summer Program; it also suggests that more personal education may be of greater importance to the academic success of urban Appalachian children than to that of children whose cultures are more object oriented.

Jerry Adams, a native Appalachian and an educator who has taught urban Appalachian students in the Cincinnati public and parochial schools for more than 20 years, gave us his interpretation of the students' desire for more personal attention:

I think it goes back many, many years, and it's been a type of myth that's been held on to. I'm not sure that the students are not given this personal attention....I think of people during the war coming to Cincinnati, people who were green from the hills, and they really weren't welcome here in greater Cincinnati, and they were told about it. And the worst thing you could have happen was to have a dumb hillbilly move into your neighborhood. And the people became very defensive and moved into their own neighborhoods with their own kind....It's been passed on to their children....These children need to be taught on the here and now—their physical needs and wants must be taken care of—"Somebody who cares enough about me not to put me down." Those teachers who really care and are personable and who care about the here and now and the demands of the day—I think those people make great strides with these kids, and that would make it...very personal. "Come to my neighborhood and see me. Come to my house. Come and eat supper with me..." Many outsiders such as the teachers are terribly frightened of doing this.

Jerry agrees with some teacher educators who recommend that we return to the practice of home visits for both preservice and in-service teachers.

So many parents are terribly frightened. So many of them are on welfare, and they are afraid if the teachers come, they will condemn them. And others feel, "If they could see how I live and that I am trying to do right, they might understand."

Jerry believes that IMPACT Home Economics, an Ohio Department of

Education program, was a very positive experience for many urban Appalachian families. Home economics teachers taught classes for one-half day and made home visits for the other half a day. In addition to teaching skills that focus on immediate needs, the IMPACT program conveyed the message that someone from the school community cared. As physical needs and wants were satisfied, teachers could begin to address the development of children's academic skills.

CULTURAL CONFLICTS AND RACIAL TENSION

You don't feel right when it's a black culture month, black this and that, but never Appalachian this or that....Blacks should be at a black school and whites should be at a white school. It's all about blacks, and you feel out of place. (Jay, 17-year-old student)

Research in Cincinnati reveals that the central city is becoming inhabited by an overwhelmingly black and Appalachian population. These residency patterns provide the context in which conflict among ethnic groups contributes to adolescents' alienation and school leaving.

As a result of busing to achieve racial integration in the Cincinnati Public Schools, most of the Summer Program participants attend Taft High School, a large, predominantly black urban school located in a low-income black neighborhood (Borman 1991). They complain that the school is foreign not only because it is not in their own neighborhood but also because their culture places them in a minority that is unrecognized by faculty members and other students. According to these youths, their sense of disenfranchisement contributes to the high dropout rate and poor school performance. Mitch, a high school senior, says:

One thing I don't like about school is that they have to send us downtown instead of going in our own neighborhood. It's harder for us to play sports and really get into school, and you hardly ever see any white people. They say it's 70–30, but it's really... more like 90–10. I don't have anything against black people, but it's most different cultures...you know, and you don't really fit in and that's why a lot of people skip school, quit, don't play sports, waste their time, and don't even try because they're going to a whole different, you know, background, and that's the reason why a lot of people mess up.

Mitch's peers in the work crew agree that he "made a lot of sense." They share similar experiences of racial tension in the classrooms and on the playing fields. Some discuss violent confrontations; others accuse black teachers of discrimination against white Appalachian students.

Belinda, a member of the girls' work crew, also referred to racial tension when making recommendations for school improvement:

I'd like to bring more white people down there because there aren't too many. There's only about 20...I guess you're so used to not being around a bunch of black people down here, and then someone rubs it in—your parents or your friends, family—that they don't like black people, and it gets to you....Because you're trying to get along better—you can get along with more people. You can learn about them, and black history—and then the teacher calls on a white person to answer the question, and they get all upset about it.

Belinda blames her own decision to leave school before graduation on racial imbalance and discrimination against low-income white Appalachians.

I dropped out for basically the same reasons others do now....How can you learn from someone who looks down on you? Like you're a piece of shit and they're above you.

Despite these perceptions, Belinda and her friends discuss a black English teacher whom they admire because she "was an equal person." They believe, however, that this teacher is an exception.

These charges of discrimination based on cultural differences echo the voices of African-American students who encounter racism in predominantly white schools. Among blacks, one response has been to flee white institutions, as evidenced by the attempts in Detroit and Atlanta to create Afrocentric schools for black children and by the 300 percent increase in black students who are fleeing white institutions to attend traditionally black colleges (Kentucky Department of Education 1991).

Ironically, these Appalachian youths would find support in the words of a black educator. Sister Thea Bowman, a consultant for Inter-Cultural Awareness, Diocese of Jackson, Mississippi, and a member of the faculty of the Black Catholic Studies Program, Xavier University, New Orleans, believes that many school faculties need greater sensitivity to the religious and cultural backgrounds of all their students. She reflects on her childhood experience as a member of "black/southern/down-home/ Gospel-oriented faith" (Bowman 1984, p. 21); she later became Catholic and attended a Catholic school in a white northern environment: "I was loved and accepted. Still, secretly, I felt very much the outsider." Bowman challenges educators to

go beyond tolerance of difference and to immerse ourselves in the multiplicity of cultures which comprise our school populations. We must learn of Black or Native American or

Hispanic or Appalachian tradition—the language, gesture, song, story, ritual—so as to help all our students become comfortable with the diversity they will surely encounter in life. (P. 23)

Cultural difference is a particularly painful issue for Appalachians. There is no consensus regarding the cultural status of the Appalachian community. Some practitioners describe Appalachians as a distinct ethnic group, like any other recognized minority. Others, like Jim Wayne Miller (1976, p. 24), conclude that

Appalachians are in no legitimate sense an ethnic group.... [They] have none of the distinguishing features of most ethnic groups—no distinguishing racial or physical features, no different language or religion. Because of this, Appalachians bear a special stigma. To have none of the marks of an "ethnic"—which serves as an explanation of different attitudes and value emphases—and yet to be so different.

In practical terms, the lack of true minority status prevents Appalachian adolescents from receiving educational and social services that frequently target specific minority populations. These youths conclude that they are both invisible and unheard by the school bureaucracy, while their black counterparts are recognized and assisted. Black culture is legitimized by the system; Appalachian culture is not. According to Jerry Adams, the resentment expressed by white Appalachian students is not at all surprising.

It's a matter of economics. You see poverty...with urban Appalachian and urban black students, and they share the same community. There's a discrimination, or they feel that it's discriminatory that one is given precedence over the other, when in actuality this black student is an ethnic minority and the Appalachian student is not. There is a great deal of resentment based upon this. What it really boils down to is really a matter of economics—coming from the same neighborhood where blacks and whites share a low-class economy. At the school the black student is given more prestige than the white student.

Attending a school in which one feels like an outsider is more than a matter of racial differences. For the children of Lower Price Hill, alienation is also a matter of geography. In order to attend high school the youths must leave their own community and travel to alien, frequently dangerous, territory.

THE NEIGHBORHOOD SCHOOL

One thing I don't like about school is that they have to send us downtown instead of going in our own neighborhood. (Mitch)

There would be less dropouts in this neighborhood and more success if we could go to high school here. (Stephen, 18-year-old student)

The issues of the neighborhood school and racial tension are related and often overlap as the Lower Price Hill youths discuss their school experiences. The importance of the neighborhood to these young people was demonstrated clearly in the investigation conducted by Borman, Mueninghoff, and Piazza (1991). A 12-year-old emphasized the youths' feelings: "To me it's the only community I've ever lived in. It's my life."

Both the boys and the girls in the Summer Program reminisce about their years in the neighborhood elementary school. Given a choice, they would forsake Taft High School, the predominantly black school "downtown," and would attend the white high school that many of their uncles and cousins had attended. Belinda recalls, "I mean, I was a leader in the fourth grade...but that's where I was stuck." Roy is enrolled in an alternative school outside the neighborhood. He likes the school because it introduces him to the world beyond the enclave where he lives and also because he believes it will "help me in the future to get a job and things." He admits, however, "I was forced to go to CAPE [Cincinnati Academy for Physical Education]. I made new friends. It's hard to leave the neighborhood. CAPE's out in the boonies. People don't mess with me and I get along."

Jay echoes the feelings of many adolescents who find themselves intimidated by the new and larger world of the high school: "You have so many buildings and so many classes and have to change so much, it gets to be too much."

The urban Appalachian youths find it especially difficult to leave a neighborhood that is "family oriented." In Mitch's words: "Everybody down here is related. Family and friends make up this community." In attempting to describe this phenomenon, Mitch begins, "Our neighborhood is like really—" and Belinda finishes the sentence for him: "...a family. We watch out for other people's kids and for each other."

Many of the parents share this desire for a school within the community. Becky, a young mother of four, recalls the demise of the neighborhood schools.

I think that if they would have kept the schools and keep the schools in the neighborhood or in a low-income area like this, a tightly knit area, like Lower Price Hill, the dropout rate would decrease a lot. I really believe this because when they started fighting them not to send our kids to Porter, I believe Roy [her son] was only in Head Start, but I went to these meetings. I attended these meetings because I knew if I stayed in this area that someday it would affect me....I know these kids. I actually believe that especially in Appalachian communities, if they had the schools closer to home, if they had the districts more or less in the same area as you lived, you would get more graduates, lessen your dropout rate. I just believe that family ties and being close to where you live is important to a lot of people.

Becky supports her argument with her own family history. Of six siblings, only two graduated from high school. Both graduates attended schools in the community; those who dropped out attended schools outside Lower Price Hill after citywide redistricting.

The youths describe an enclave consisting of such tightly woven interfamily relationships that kin share responsibility for the discipline of each other's children. For the teenagers this situation is both supportive and intrusive. Mitch points out that "if you're ever in trouble, you'll have the whole neighborhood in back of you." At the same time, this closeness interferes with behaviors such as drug use, despite easy access to drugs. Stephen, one member of the group, claimed that the parents themselves were the major users and abusers of drugs, particularly marijuana. The following conversation describes the obstacles to drug use in the community:

Mitch: See, really, it's hard to get anything in this neighborhood because of the parents.

Belinda: Everybody knows everybody's kids. You're not going to give somebody else's kids shit [drugs] unless you want trouble.

Stephen: [That's] A lot of bull—money talks; bullshit walks. The kids are scared their parents will find out and they will find out. Most of the kids are not hooked on pot and drugs—it's the parents. The kids use mostly wine coolers. Like if someone knows your parents and you've got the money for stuff, and [if] you use anything, someone will tell your parents. The old women sit out in front—they'll see ya.

Mitch: They'll tell your mom and hardly finish a crossword puzzle.

Although these youths claim that drug use is virtually nonexistent, some spoke knowledgeably about the price, quality, and sources of marijuana and about the availability of "pills" and amphetamines in the neighborhood. The availability of "downers" was attributed to the presence of the public health clinic in the neighborhood. Clinic staff members were viewed as dispensing drugs carelessly into the community. Nonetheless, drinking is the most widespread abusive activity in this group of teenagers. Larry Redden, a social worker, said about the hard drugs: "Crack is virtually no more. It's gone." Although still available in African-American neighborhoods, it is rejected by these youths who see it as part of a "black style" that they do not find attractive.

The girls' neighborhood experience differs somewhat from the boys'. Among the girls, being on the streets with the guys is a source of entertainment and fun, although such behavior also exposes them to gang violence, drinking, and drug use. These girls, however, spoke of avoiding or being protected from involvement with drugs and alcohol by concerned parents and other adults in the neighborhood. Such protectiveness often caused frustration. One of the girls talked about her "experience with drug use," as she called it:

I had an experience with drug use....I did it last year—well, when I was doing my senior year. I snuck away with some friends of mine up the street. I mean, we'd sit right there in front of the bar and some guy...said, "You don't want to mess up right now"—talking to me...[that way] since it was my senior year. He said if he saw me doing it again, he'd go tell my parents. And then one of my other friends told me to come down here and talk to Fred [a counselor at the Urban Appalachian Council], and he gave me this long lecture.

As young women, they perceived that they were more severely restricted in their behavior by parents and neighbors who were anxious that the girls avoid early pregnancy. In comparing herself to her brother, Bonnie remarked:

My father is harder on me than on my brother. I mean, I can see why because he doesn't want me to go out there—me being a girl—I mean, you see all these girls doing the same thing. Someone's 14 with a baby. He doesn't want me to end up like that. So I'm living with a man who doesn't want me to mess up.

Parental strategies that aim at sequestering young women are not limited to urban Appalachian families, of course. Such strategies are prevalent in paternalistic ethnic cultures. Although these strategies perhaps are effective in the short run, they can deprive young women of opportunities (1) to participate in community life, (2) to have experiences that prepare them for adulthood, and (3) to adopt a less passive orientation to life. One notable aspect of the interviews with these young women was the emphasis on their role as companions to the boys, who initiated fights, drinking bouts, and other street action while they simply went along as passive observers. The role of passive observer is not consistent with either academic or career-related achievement.

The use of drugs and alcohol in the neighborhood spills over into school. Kids who smoke marijuana persist in school if they "focus their mind on school" and use pot only occasionally. Pouring beer or whiskey into coke bottles and slipping it into school, an activity undertaken by "a whole bunch of guys," was reported by the girls.

Despite their objections to the watchful eyes of their mothers and grandmothers, the Summer Program participants perceive the neighborhood to be a safe place, a place where they are respected and not considered "hillbillies" or "white trash." Leaving this home ground is threatening—both to their physical well-being, because they encounter rival gangs, and to their self-image, because they feel "put down" by school staff members who do not understand their culture. Although the youths suggest a return to the simpler days of attending the neighborhood school, in the long run they would not benefit from continued isolation from the larger society in which they live. Jerry Adams comments as follows on their wish to remain secluded:

I think part of that is enculturation. When I think back to the parents who were here for years and years, as long as they were with their own, they felt comfortable....To a certain extent, when I talk to some Appalachians they still feel that schools are against them and don't understand them....If they go outside their own community, they will run into those people who will hate them and despise them and will treat them as a low-class minority....In the neighborhood school they felt safe. They knew the teacher; they knew the principal. They could make the home visits, and it was a safety factor that was built in and that can't exist forever. The same thing happens down in the hills. When I taught children down there and children had to leave community schools and go to junior high and high schools, you saw the tremendous number of dropouts there, too....That's where we need to do a lot of education to get these kids ready....You have to handpick teachers who love kids....Make sure that there's some transitional counseling or guidance for these kids on how to succeed and get along. First, get the families involved....It will be very difficult with their attitude.

With an increase in gang-related activities, the perception of the neighborhood as a protective fortress also emerges. Boys and girls alike view life in the neighborhood as both dangerous and boring. The boys talked about gangs of more affluent white youths from Price Hill and elsewhere who come into the neighborhood, particularly on the weekends. Gangs with colorful names like OGs (Original Gangsters), Miami Boys, C-Town, Cincy Boys, and the Mod Squad operate according to a "policy" designed to terrify those they encounter. Betsy, the Youth Program leader, a long-term resident of Lower Price Hill and mother of one of the boys, said of the gangs:

Their policy is to find you by yourself and beat the shit out of you. They never fight
one-on-one. They keep the odds on their side. They use guns, Mace. You name it, they
got it.

Lower Price Hill youths do not view gang membership as attractive.
Nonetheless, two of the boys wearing western-style kerchiefs declared
amidst much hooting that they were the "bandanna bastards." Although
gang activity centers around cars (as opposed to motorcycles) and is
motivated by claims on girls living in the neighborhood, both of which
interest male Youth Program participants, gang membership is shunned
primarily for three reasons: (1) "They're always fighting" (Mitch); (2)
"They want to be black" (Stephen); and (3) "You don't need a gang
down here to be supported" (Betsy).

Despite these protestations, gang activity continued to increase
during the fall of 1991. By early December, television news crews were
on the scene in Lower Price Hill with members of the OGs and special
police units assigned to quell the rise of gang violence in the neighborhood (ABC, December 5, 1991). In light of the discussion of racial
tensions, it is interesting to note that the Lower Price Hill gangs include
both black and white members. According to one white youth, a
particular black member "motivates [the other members]....He's a tough
kid."

The foregoing discussion of the multiple meanings of *neighborhood*
to urban Appalachian youths underlines the need for educational
institutions to build on community strengths. The Appalachian
community can become a powerful ally or an equally powerful adversary
of the school system. Without the support of the neighborhood,
educational reform is doomed to failure.

RECOMMENDATIONS FOR CHANGE

The lives of the Lower Price Hill youths demonstrate clearly that
current educational programs and policies fail to adequately address
poverty, alienation, and racism. Even more discouraging, perhaps,
current reform efforts do not begin to address the academic failures of
urban Appalachian adolescents because they do not fully consider the
social context in which that failure occurs. Change must be comprehensive and systemic, not piecemeal. Children who arrive at school with a
background that includes hunger, violence, drugs, lack of health
insurance, and cultural prejudice cannot be expected to function well

academically. Despite federal recognition that children must start school "ready to learn," precious little action is directed toward that goal in Lower Price Hill and other communities like it.

The following recommendations are not exhaustive; they are conclusions based on our conversations with the at-risk youths who spoke with us at the Urban Appalachian Council.

Federal Guidelines

Federal and state definitions of *minority* must be expanded to include Appalachians. Urban Appalachian youths and their families currently are penalized for their cultural differences but do not qualify for most programs designed to assist minorities in their struggle to achieve the "American dream." There is no safety net for the invisible urban Appalachian adolescent.

Defining Appalachians as a recognized minority group will accomplish three distinct goals related to school achievement. First, it will allow them to qualify for the kind of programs that provide for the daily "needs and wants" (Adams 1991) that must be satisfied before they can concentrate on cognitive issues.

Second, as members of a recognized minority group, adolescent Appalachians can channel the energy currently spent on resentment toward and competition with other recognized minorities to focus creatively and energetically on their own priorities. As the work force becomes increasingly diverse, the Appalachian youths' unwillingness to mix with outsiders becomes increasingly dysfunctional. Their self-imposed isolation militates against success in high school, college and/or job training programs, and the workplace.

Third, new definitions will support continued research on these youths with the collection of more complete data on school leaving and academic achievement; such data are collected as a matter of course in large survey studies such as the National Assessment of Educational Progress (NAEP). In particular, we need to collect and analyze data that will yield additional information on these youths' specific strengths and weaknesses and allow us to formulate answers to some crucial questions. For example, why is there such a disparity between their mathematical and their verbal skills? Which factors contribute to the academic success of those urban Appalachian students who do "make it"? How can these success factors be translated into assistance for all at-risk Appalachian students?

Education of Teachers

Teachers, both pre-service and in-service, must be aware of the subtle interplay among variables of culture, academic achievement, and students' perceptions of equality and fairness. Initial efforts to improve teachers' preparation for effectively addressing cultural diversity in the classroom have not been promising. McDiarmid (1990) conducted a four-year study of persons who received training designed specifically to prepare them to teach a variety of learners. He concluded that presentations appear to have little effect on how teachers think about these issues, and he raises questions about the content and the pedagogy of multicultural programs. Both researchers and participants found an inherent weakness in programs that attempted to address diversity of students by sharing information about cultural similarities and differences. As one participant stated:

The problem is that we're told all the time that this is a group and that we're supposed to look upon their cultural background. So every time that I get an insight from somebody about [culturally different learners], that automatically translates in my mind, and I think it would be very difficult for it not to be...a stereotype....So, I think that...what I've got to do is somehow take what I'm getting here [in this course] about this multicultural experience and forget about it. (McDiarmid 1990, p. 17)

Despite such lackluster, even counterproductive efforts, an entire industry has emerged in response to issues of diversity. Further research is essential to identify both curricula and pedagogy needed to prepare teachers to meet the needs of learners who are different from themselves. Initial efforts must focus on the "success stories." What characteristics or behaviors distinguish the black English teacher who was considered "an equal person" from her less positively regarded colleagues? Another teacher, Mr. P, was described by one of the boys as

a hell of a teacher. He would get on your case...and he'll let you know what he's doing. But then you also like him for the way he teaches....Some teachers you feel good about. You kind of have to have a teacher who will push you. Like to make you do the work and not just sit there.

What can we learn from these effective teachers that we can apply to the professional preparation of all teachers? Teacher education can be improved by acting on what we know already from the research. We know, for example, that attitudes are rarely changed by lectures about the need for changing our attitudes. Experiences, however, can be powerful means of altering belief systems. Home visits and other experiences that bring both preservice and in-service teachers into close contact with their students outside the classroom not only may transform the teachers' perspectives but also will convey the concern inherent in "more personal" schooling.

Links between Neighborhood and School

The theme of the neighborhood as refuge has important implications for social service and educational policy and delivery systems that affect urban Appalachians. Larry Redden, a social worker serving the urban Appalachian community, noted that schools have become more cynical:

The community pays attention to the minority group that's the established minority group. The board of education…even though they realize there is another subminority group, or whatever you call it, out there with problems just as large, it's still invisible and not really anything is happening. In our city today, we've got maybe a thousand [social service] agencies and organizations in the network, and the targeted population is the black community.

A proliferation of agencies with overlapping functions is an acknowledged problem in all urban centers. Indeed, the United Way nationally has begun efforts to consolidate and coordinate social service delivery. Larry spoke of his vision for improving the system:

Like any other social worker that's going to be here for a long time, I've got the perfect answer. But it makes too much sense and, for that reason, it probably wouldn't be considered. Bureaucracies tend to establish themselves in making things as difficult as possible. They pride themselves on…making it so difficult you don't even know what they're doing. It's really [evident] when a person goes for a service at a certain place and gets herded to another place and so on. What you need is a multipurpose center within the communities themselves. We've got 48, 49 communities in the city, and we need multipurpose centers that serve each and every one of those communities, doing the same kind of things for each and every one of them. We've got the facilities…to do that.

Larry's plan is simple. He believes that neighborhood-based services, centrally located in the targeted community and housed in the neighborhood school, hold the promise for the service delivery and responsibility to the community that currently are lacking in the highly bureaucratized and overlapping social service delivery system. The school is a perfect locale for these services:

In each community, there's a school building. During the winter, school goes from 8:00 A.M. to 3:00 P.M. After the afternoon is over, social services could take over. The people of that community could use that school as their center which all activity would flow around. You could have your counselors, social workers, and recreation people in each one. It would eliminate the necessity of building all these other big building[s]....You've got people out there working with people—one-on-one. The people would be in the community, so they could get to know where the problems are and get to know who the kids are, who the adults are, where the problems are, and they could have their hands on full-time. This could happen year-round. In the summertime, the school would open as a multipurpose center. Almost every high school in the city has a swimming pool. You would eliminate the necessity of having a swimming pool in the parks.

Everything is all mixed up the way it is now. It could all be combined. The community council could have community input because the councils could work out of this school; your volunteers could set up by triggering programs. If they stop and think about it, they could do almost anything they wanted. It's right there on the spot in the community, and it can be controlled.

According to Larry, present arrangements for such service delivery perhaps are seen most clearly in the operation of the parochial schools because parochial schools are rooted directly in the local community and tend to be responsive.

There's a structure there that helps because people feel that they own that structure. It's their school, their church, their whole everything. You have poor people in the schools, too. Once people can get together, they can help themselves and work on those kinds of things. That's the closest you can come to it now, and it could be done better. Rather than the city funding that money to a special recreation program which has it's [own] administration, they'd just have one administration to do the hiring of people for certain areas. You'd be cutting budgets down, cutting everything. The public school system doesn't have to pay double for heating and the like...and they would be saving money. It could work. You have people out there who like to do funding, and you could have those people work on that for the school. In each school you've got an auditorium, so they could put on community plays, events, and so on. But unfortunately, you've [also] got bureaucracy.

Larry's observations make a good deal of sense for the organization and delivery of social and educational services. Similar programs are beginning to emerge in the Commonwealth of Kentucky as part of the Kentucky Education Reform Act. Although they are not necessarily located in school buildings, family and youth resource centers are providing health and social services to families and adolescents as part of the education reform. The Kentucky legislature recognizes that basic survival needs must be met before students can excel in the classroom.

Adequate provision of social services is the foundation for improved academic performance. The neighborhood-school link, however, must extend beyond those services. In communities across the nation, educators are combining classroom work with service or social action projects that build on local circumstances and teachers' insights. Nathan and Kielsmeier (1991) list some examples.

In Salt Lake City, fourth-through-sixth-grade students have been responsible for the cleanup of a hazardous waste site, the passage of two new environmental laws, the planting of hundreds of trees, and the completion of a number of other neighborhood improvements. The families of the students...have the lowest per-capita income in Salt Lake City, and the students themselves aren't unusually gifted or articulate. (P. 740)

In the South Bronx, students at South Bronx Regional High School are working with a community organization to restore a building that will provide housing for the homeless, some of whom are members of the students' own families. Other examples include a day care center in Brooks County, Georgia, a playground planned and implemented by a group of five- to nine-year-olds, and a consumer program in which inner-city public school students successfully resolved more than 75 percent of the 350 cases submitted to them by adults. In each example, young people are learning by solving real problems in their own communities.

The appeal of such programs is articulated most clearly by Mitch, a member of the boys' work crew, who had graduated from the unique public school alternative program offered by the Inland Waterways Academy. Before enrolling in the program, he had been a discipline problem and was skipping classes. This behavior stopped when he began to attend the academy.

That school was different....The classes were small, and the teacher had time to give everyone the special attention they needed and help you with your stuff and teach you, and you could see what you could do.

"Seeing what you could do" is possible in a program with a limited enrollment, which focuses on a specific set of skills and allows participants to apply those skills in the actual work environment in which they are required. Education reform for urban Appalachian youths can combine the strong neighborhood affiliation with the desire to see "what you could do." Ken Nelson, a Minnesota state representative and an advocate of learning from service, recommends that we shift our focus from labels such as "at-risk" to "youth potential, youth strengths, youth participation, and contributions" (Nelson 1988, p. 5).

Too many efforts directed toward the academic achievement of low-socioeconomic urban youth have focused on "fixing the kids." Our conversations with the Summer Program participants suggest that the schooling itself must be "fixed" to address the unique concerns of Appalachian adolescents. Their successes tell us that the social climate of the school not only must be personal in the sense of small class size and individual attention but also must respect their Appalachian cultural heritage. It must allow them to learn with dignity. Successful educational institutions are tied closely to the community and draw strength from a solid parent network. Educational research supports the contentions of these youths. It is time for educational reformers to hear their voices and act on their recommendations.

12

Readin', Writin', and Route 23:
A Road to Economic
but Not Educational Success
Johanna S. DeStefano

The dark ribbon of the road, stained by countless dripping oil pans and leaky transmissions, meanders north to Columbus, Toledo, and Detroit, where tens of thousands of drivers and their passengers hoped they would find better economic times. It wasn't the "Promised Land" so many black folks thought Chicago was, after World War I, because it wasn't home. But up north, U.S. Route 23 was lined with jobs.

Starting at the Atlantic Ocean in northern Florida and skirting the Okefenokee Swamp in southern Georgia, the road finally peters out at the Mackinac Strait at the top of Michigan, without entering the wastes of the Upper Peninsula. That frozen area used Route 23, too, in the opposite direction. Its people, mostly Finns and other Scandinavians, traveled south to the vast manufacturing belt of southern Michigan where the iron they had mined poured into the cars of America.

The automotive plants in Columbus and Toledo, along with other heavy and light manufacturing, were the economic engines driving the good times. These plants drew Appalachians living in the hills of eastern Kentucky and Tennessee and western West Virginia up Route 23. They had a saying: if you wanted to make yourself and yours a better life than you could down home, you'd better get some readin' and writin', and then get up Route 23. Some black folks, sharecroppers who'd been kicked off the land, had picked up Route 23 in Georgia; that's how Dick's father reached Columbus.

Tom, Dick, and Harry work at one of the automotive plants still producing parts in Columbus. The factory used to employ more than 4,000 workers on the lines, operating the heavy presses that stamp out the parts. With almost 1 million square feet under the roof, ghosts from the heyday of mass production fill the dim corners and vast empty areas, circling around the diminished islands that still shake the floor and destroy the hearing while pushing out the auto body parts.

Those workers who are left number about 1,600, have at least 15 years of seniority on the job, and are mostly urban Appalachian, sometimes as far back as three or four generations. They are among the decreasing numbers of urban Appalachians mentioned by Borman (1991) who work as craftspersons and operatives, remnants of factory workers from the 1940s into the 1970s, when generally little or no experience or training was required. Because they are employed, however, they are not part of the more general picture painted by Borman (1991) when she notes that "many third and fourth generation urban Appalachian families remain isolated and out of work" (p. 8).

About 5 percent of the remaining line workers are African-American, including Dick. Virtually all of the others come either from the Appalachian counties of southeastern Ohio or from south of Broad Street or U.S. Route 40, the old National Road.

Broad Street also is the main east-west street in Columbus, bisecting it almost evenly between north and south. It still marks the boundary between the South and the North Midland dialects, although more so in the past than now. South Midland is spoken by most of the Appalachians who followed Route 23 to Columbus, as well as by those who live in Grove City to the immediate south of Columbus. Grove City, however, has been affected over time by the North Midland band. South of Broad Street, people say "boosh," "poosh," and "warsh." North of Broad Street, they say "bush," "push," and "wash." Most of the differences are phonological, although some syntactic markers still are present and carry a class stigma. These include "He done it" and "I ain't got none." Whatever the forms may be now, it is clear that "much of Ohio, especially, speaks with an Appalachian accent." (Maloney 1981, p. 169)

These "boosh"- and "warsh"-using workers at the "BodyWorks" plant are represented by the United Auto Workers (UAW), one of the strongest unions in the country. Although smaller than in the past, it is still a formidable force among the Big Three automakers. Consequently, these workers have about as much job security as is possible in the private sector, given the threat of continued plant closings. As a result, they can count on the average annual pay levels of around $35,000 far more strongly than most manufacturing workers can count on either pay or a job. This figure is more than four times the $7,788 reported by Borman (1991) as the average annual family income among the urban Appalachians of Lower Price Hill, an enclaved neighborhood in Cincinnati, and also is above average nationwide.

Economically, then, Tom and Harry, the two urban Appalachian hourly employees, enjoy continuing success of the kind that is no longer widely prevalent—based on lower skills and higher wages rather than on the increasingly dominant situation in which higher skills are required for lower wages. In the working class, the two men undoubtedly are considered quite successful, with their well-paying, relatively stable jobs, their homes, their hobbies, and their intact, two-parent families. For some Appalachians, the ride up Route 23 clearly brought greater prosperity and possibly "a better life," at least in economic terms, for several generations.

Yet "a better life" includes more than economic aspects. As Obermiller reminds us, "Research should include both personal (value expressive) and psychological indicators as well as the standard socioeconomic and political indicators among Appalachians. Standard social indicators give only a one-sided view of lives which are often rich and complex" (1981, p. 17). These factors and others, such as certain forms of educational achievement are part of the definition of a life and part of its complexity; they are part of the lives of both Tom and Harry.

Both men feel that something is missing from their lives, that somehow the better life has eluded them. For Tom, it's "readin'"; for Harry, it's "writin'". So although they no longer fit the "image of poverty" that Precourt (1983) describes, thus escaping the tribal stigma of race (Goffman in Precourt 1983, p. 6) and being able to "swim in the mainstream," they still feel stigmatized. They suffer the "blemishes of individual character" (Goffman in Precourt 1983, p. 8). Tom, who couldn't read when he entered a work force literacy program at BodyWorks, adeptly hid this deficiency from his fellow workers and bosses. His various intelligent, sometimes brilliant, subterfuges reveal his terrible fear of being found "blemished." Harry was so ashamed of his self-perceived lack of ability to spell that he had long ago stopped writing anything to anyone, on or off the job, at great personal cost to himself. While the literacy program was available at BodyWorks, Harry finally came in secretly to try to rid himself of the blemish of being essentially a nonwriter.

Educational success, including some basic literacy skills, does not necessarily coincide with better economic times for Appalachians. As this author (DeStefano 1991) noted, Appalachian students' dropout rates in Columbus schools are the highest of any ethnic group. Also, my research with "Tom" as a first-grade pupil (not the Tom of BodyWorks but a first-generation Appalachian in Columbus) found that he was repeating the first grade because of his "lack of development of reading skills" (DeStefano, Pepinsky and Sanders 1982). Furthermore, in at least one school, all of the urban Appalachian boys in the first grade were repeating that grade except two, both of whom were on Ritalin. The difficulty was perceived mostly as lack of necessary reading skills, based in part on spotty school attendance. This pattern, which often demonstrates great disruptions, unfortunately is not uncommon in the group but goes largely undocumented.

The current study of Tom's and Harry's literacy skills is among the first about urban Appalachian adults. It is also among the first case studies of adults' specific reading and writing difficulties. Researchers who have concentrated on adult issues typically have hardly looked beyond demographics, projections of how many persons are reading at what levels, wholesale assessment issues, and so on. Individual learners and their personal struggles with print also have been largely forgotten in the political rhetoric about how the American work force is illiterate and not skilled enough and in the battle for funds for programs. Meanwhile, the parameters of the problem, the needs, and the definition of a literate adult in a postindustrial society are not yet understood.

METHODOLOGY

A development and demonstration project established an educational center where plant employees could receive workplace instruction in literacy and basic skills. This project provided me with the opportunity to conduct case studies of Tom and Harry. With Tom, I was an observer and interviewer; with Harry, I was a participant observer, serving as his spelling instructor.

These case studies (along with a study of Dick, the urban African-American worker at the plant) are part of a series of "Tom, Dick, and Harry" studies in which the participants' ages range from three years to the midforties and early fifties. The goal is to collect cross-sectional data on language and literacy experiences and usage across much of the life span of urban Appalachian, urban African-American, and mainstream males living in Columbus, Ohio.

At BodyWorks, I interviewed Tom over a 6-month period. Our interview began after he had made some progress in learning to read and was more willing to talk with others about why he was coming to work with one of the teachers in the workplace literacy program. The interviews and the samples of oral reading were concluded in December 1991, when Tom had been in the program for almost 12 months. Only then was it possible to ask him to read aloud into a tape recorder, not because he had not wanted anyone to know before then but because he had lacked confidence. After several months in the program, Tom decided to "come out of the closet" regarding his lack of ability to read.

He learned to explain to people that he had a problem but was "becoming a reader."

It was possible to collect more data on Tom than on Harry because Tom was officially part of the program. He had been transferred into a position that allowed him to spend his entire work shift in the learning center as an aide when he wasn't working at learning to read. The data include not only the extensive interview but also interviews with his teacher and his supervisor. Samples of his reading aloud are also included. Thus, his profile as a beginning reader can reflect his immediate superior's evaluation of changes (if any) in his work habits.

Harry was actively involved with me in spelling work over a little more than two months, from early September to mid-November 1991. During that period, I met with him at least weekly for two- to three-hour instructional sessions. I served as his instructor because I have extensive background in American English traditional orthography and in spelling instruction with more advanced students. I kept notes from interviews with Harry and from the lessons themselves, although I did no taping because of his concern about confidentiality. Harry was extremely concerned that fellow workers, supervisors, engineers—anyone—would learn that he had spelling problems. Thus, his learner profile does not include the interviews that were possible with Tom.

This profile, however, includes an intake interview prepared for collecting background data and learners' perceptions regarding spelling as a literacy problem. It also includes a profile of learning styles adapted especially for use in the project, a reading-aloud selection from Harry's workplace reading material, a close assessment, and a Gap assessment. The two latter items are specific reading assessment instruments; both use text from the workplace. I created the Gap as a means of obtaining more detailed knowledge of a reader's text comprehension. I administered the various reading measures in order to find out whether Harry had a receptive competence problem (e.g., reading) as well as a productive competence problem (namely, spelling) because the two might have some connection, depending on the nature of his specific problems.

FINDINGS

Tom

Tom is a 43-year-old urban Appalachian male with 15 years' seniority at BodyWorks. During those years, he has worked on a variety of stamping presses and also has packed the finished parts. Even though Tom was a complete nonreader when he entered the program at the learning center, with a word recognition vocabulary of about 20 words, and possessed only the most rudimentary mathematical skills, he had a high school diploma from a small city school system just south of Columbus. Thus, his family lived in a suburban setting, although it was a working-class town believed to be populated almost exclusively by urban Appalachians. Yet Tom was passed through the grades without developing the abilities necessary for success in school. In high school he was part of a vocational education program that allowed the students to work half of each day during the school week. Thus, during his two final years in high school, he was not in the school building for half of the school year. When he was present, he spent his time in various shop classes.

In elementary and middle school, Tom was passed quietly from grade to grade, largely because "I didn't give 'em no trouble." That observation is probably accurate because he certainly could not have done any regular schoolwork, taken tests, or really participated in the educational aspects of schooling.

Because of his lack of basic abilities in reading, writing, and arithmetic, Tom essentially could do only manual labor. Fortunately for him, his father was employed at BodyWorks, and so was able to have him hired, but only on the second try. The first time Tom applied, about 10 years before he was finally hired, the vision test, which was part of the initial screening process, was made up of words that the subject was supposed to call out, rather than letters. Because Tom couldn't recognize the words—clear evidence of a reading problem—he failed the vision test and was not hired. In fact, his vision is good; he still does not wear corrective lenses. On his second try, the vision test had been changed to consist of common letter patterns of various sizes. Because Tom could recognize letters, he passed this test and was hired.

Since starting his program at the learning center, Tom has been an "all-purpose operator" on a line that manufactures the entire auto body part from start to finish. In this departure from typical line work in which each worker performs only a few operations, the workers are organized in teams with all the machinery necessary to complete the entire part among themselves. This move to synchronous manufacturing is one of the changes sweeping the industry, impelled by fear of Japanese auto manufacturers and by the use of Japanese work configurations in the hope of enhancing the company's competitive position in the market.

To become an all-purpose operator, one of the official job designations in the plant, each employee must take a training program and be certified. The training includes manuals and paper-and-pencil work, which are provided by staff of the plant training department. Somehow, Tom passed through the program without having to do any reading or writing, most likely on the basis of oral input, watching demonstrations, and hands-on, on-the-job learning (probably his major mode of learning). He obtained his certification and moved to the specially configured line, where he became a team boss for a period of time.

According to his supervisor (his immediate superior), Tom is one of the most effective operators in all the teams under his supervision. Tom figures out when the team must "jump" from one machine to the next in order to produce its quota of parts during a shift. In this complicated process, the operator must understand how long it takes a given machine to stamp out a certain number of parts, and then must coordinate that knowledge with the manufacturing rates of the other machines on the line rates. If a team is to "make their money" during their shift—that is, fill their quota—the end result must be a certain number of finished parts below a certain defect rate. If the parts are not produced, the operators' wages suffer because they are paid by piecework. Above all, Tom wants to "make his money." Tom is described by his supervisor as a quality worker despite his lack of basic skills. In fact, the supervisor indicated that literacy wasn't necessary on Tom's job or for doing a good job. Tom, however, could not move beyond being an operator in BodyWorks. He has had several opportunities to be promoted off the line, but each time he has refused, largely, he says, because he couldn't do the necessary paperwork. Now, because of his relatively low seniority in the plant, he has some fear of being transferred to a job that requires use of the computer, either directly in the manufacturing process or for quality control through computerized measurement of parts.

Language and Literacy Interview

1. *"What made you decide to come to our workplace literacy program?"*

Tom said it took him a long time to make the decision: he was "scared" about coming and deeply ashamed of his inability to read. He said that his pride prevented him from coming for months because he'd kept his inability to read a secret at the plant. His wife, however, who is literate and works for the state of Ohio, kept urging him to try it, so he came in about five months after the program started. He said, "If it was up to me, I probably wouldn't have learned to read [he is not yet an independent reader], 'cause if you never have it, you never miss it." Yet it was also clear that he did "miss it." This ambivalence continued to surface throughout his work in the program.

The "blemish of individual character" surfaced when Tom talked about being illiterate in a basically literate world. He called himself a con artist, referring to the strategies he used to hide this blemish. For example, when his foreman brings him something to read, Tom says, "My hands are all dirty. I can't hold it. Read it to me." If someone asks him, "Did you read about X in the paper?" he says, "I didn't have time. Tell me about it." Sometimes he takes some items home for his wife to read to him. As he put it, he'd spent his life talking others into reading for him.

2. *"Has your attitude toward learning changed since you've been coming to the center?"*

Tom said that his attitude toward life, not only toward learning, had changed. In the past, he had felt much more defensive, "afraid to be in crowds 'cause I couldn't read." Evidently, this comment referred to his expressed fear that he might have been expected to read something. Now he tells people that he's "becoming a reader." He also participates more in team discussions on the job, and served as team boss; in this position, he had to take other workers' complaints to the supervisor.

3. *"If you could read and write better and do math better, do you think you could be more productive on your job?"*

Tom didn't think so, and neither did his supervisor. In this connection, however, he had been asked to move up in rank but had to refuse promotion because he couldn't perform the duties requiring literacy skills. Also, as mentioned before, Tom lived in fear of having to take a job among the increasing number of jobs that involved more skills than he had.

4. *"If BodyWorks gave you more educational opportunities, would you use them?"*

Tom said he would do so but that his first goal was learning to read. He then described the role, whether realistic or not, that he thinks reading could play in his life. First, he said he'd missed a great deal in life because he couldn't read, such as general information, history, and geography. (His teacher confirmed that Tom doesn't seem to know a great deal about current events, local issues, or much beyond the daily experiences of his life.) For example, Tom feels that he can't carry on a sports conversation with his two sons because he can't read the sports section of the newspaper. Then he said, "I've worked second shift all my life to stay away from my boys"; he couldn't bear the thought of them seeing how much he didn't know. He ended with, "It's a lonely world."

For whatever reason, Tom has decided that his inability to read is at the root of many of his family communication problems and problems of self-esteem. At this point, literacy researchers know little about how reading problems interact with self-concept, self-esteem, and interpersonal relationships. Perhaps Tom's statements afford a glimmer of insight into these unknown interactions.

5. *"Are the experiences at this center different from the learning experiences you had in school?"*

Tom's answer was a resounding yes. For him, two outstanding characteristics were the personal instruction in the one-on-one learning situation and the instructor's attention, which helped him concentrate on his instruction. He said that in school he could slough off as long as he didn't make trouble and sat in the back. In the learning center, his instructor "kept him on his toes." Another major advantage in his mind was that he was in the program by choice. He said that he had been forced to go to school, so he had a "bad attitude because they were making me do it."

Another difference was Tom's deep anger about his school experiences, especially toward the teachers who failed to teach him to read. He stated adamantly that the first five grades were the "most important time" in a child's life, when the teachers "have got to help them learn to read." He said, "I'd like to take away the reading rights of some of those teachers and see how they feel."

Evidently, Tom was promoted through the grades without much diagnosis or special instruction, although he mentioned having two special reading teachers for a short period sometime during his years in school. "That didn't last long," he commented.

Tom felt strongly that he should have had the help of a reading specialist from the very beginning and referred to hearing problems he had had in the first grade. He said, "I probably couldn't hear, so by third or fourth grade, it was too late." In reality, he probably was not extremely hard of hearing, but his ear infections distracted him. If one has other difficulties initially, they compound one another. In addition, he was diagnosed at a reading clinic as having, as he puts it, "some kind of lexia—some big word." *Dyslexia*, the word he meant, is a portmanteau term that is not very revealing but often refers, among other things, to difficulties in sound-letter correspondence. Tom did not understand that sounds in words correspond to written letters. He also tends to reverse letters and words: *saw* becomes *was*, *ps* becomes *qs*, *bs* becomes *ds*, and vice versa.

Thus, Tom is convinced that he could have, and should have, learned to read, beginning in the first grade, and that he did not learn essentially because of poor teaching. He summed up his 12 years in school with, "It was a big waste. I lost 12 years of my life I'll never get back. And they were some of my best."

6. *"Do you find reading easy or difficult? Writing and spelling easy or difficult? Expressing yourself orally to others?"* (Tom now had been in the program almost a year, so it was important to gauge his feelings toward these activities.)

Reading. Tom responded that reading is both easy and difficult for him: "It's still hard, but some of it ain't as hard." He categorizes as the easy part at sight, such as words that he recognizes: *the, it, to,* and *for*. He said he didn't know them before he started instruction, which is one of the marks of a nonreader.

Tom finds it difficult, however, to make sound-letter correspondences. In other words, he has trouble sounding out words. This problem is understandable because letters can and do represent different sounds in different words in English. One difficulty for Tom is the *g* in *laugh*. He has little trouble with the correspondences in words such as *go* and *get*, but he does not yet remember that the *gh* combination symbolizes the /f/ sound in *laugh* (/laf/) and is part of the larger pattern including *cough, tough,* and others.

Tom still is largely at the stage of thinking that each letter must have a sound, except for the few so-called silent letters he knows about, such as the final e in single-syllable words such as *fate*. Strictly speaking, the *e* is part of the grapheme vowel-consonant *e* for the tense vowel in a word such as *fate*. Tom has yet to make these sound-letter correspondence patterns an automatic part of his word recognition system.

Tom clearly is establishing certain habits that are novel and not easy, in part because he performs some reversals of letters and words. This tendency to reverse is not his main problem, however, and probably was not a major contributing factor to his failure to learn to read in elementary school.

Another reason why reading is hard for Tom is that (as he points out), he's never done it before. One of his major goals is to be able to sit down and read a book, in a sense to join the literate society he sees around him but from which he has been barred all his life. Sometimes, however, he makes comments such as, "Right now, I could take it or leave it [meaning reading]. If the center closed, I'd never do it again." This ambivalence characterizes Tom's feelings about learning to read and could cause him to stop trying to learn when the program closes and his instructor leaves.

If Tom were to stop at this stage of his literacy development, undoubtedly he would not become a reader because he does not approach being an independent reader. When reading on his own, unaided by his instructor, he becomes bogged down in word recognition. In view of his small sight vocabulary and his lack of automatic word recognition skills, it is understandable that Tom dislikes reading on his own. His instructor supplies the word when he encounters trouble and also gives him clues to help him untangle himself.

The following examples show his decoding level of skill. First, in the sentence "Everyone agrees on the biggest problem," Tom was unable to read *everyone*; he read it as *English.*

Second, Tom read the sentence "Rachel says, 'I want to know English so that I can understand the news' " as "Rachel says, 'I want to know English so that I can use...d...uset...dah...use...en...us it...dah... n...n...short e...neh...neh...double us...in...war...in...neh...next... next—so that I can use it? Duh...n...short es eh...en...I...I...want to know wuh...how...double u's wuh...what...what...I want to know... double u's wuh...write...double us wuh...short a sound... wat...wat's...what's going on.' " His word recognition skills broke down completely on *understand* and also on *news*. In fact, he tends to have difficulties with many words of two or more syllables.

Writing and Spelling. At first, Tom defined writing as copying. He said he had no problem writing, that he could write as fast as anyone. For him, writing was not a process of putting his thoughts down on paper but of reproducing something that someone else had written without his processing it in any way. Later he began to describe "bringing it out of his head" as very difficult for him, largely, he said, because of his problems with spelling. He feels compelled to spell every word "correctly" and does not seem to be willing to approximate. Because Tom approaches spelling through the same laborious sounding-out process as he uses with word recognition (which leads to errors), he finds writing both difficult and tedious. Not surprisingly, his output is minimal and he often resorts to copying.

Tom said spelling is hard for him because "the English language is so messed up." He is confused and frustrated by the lack of what are (to him) clear phoneme-grapheme correspondences. Tom asks why certain letters appear and others do not and is angry that we receive so many words from so many different languages without changing their spellings. This last piece of information came to him through me; I worked with classes in the center on spelling, including word origin. Obviously, Tom listened in, although he did not participate in the classes.

Tom as a Literate Worker

At this point, Tom finds reading very laborious and extremely time-consuming. Sometimes he feels it isn't worth the effort; at other times, he is pleased with his progress, such as his increasing sight vocabulary. Tom said:

I'm a beginner. I'm learning from the ground up. It's a whole new ball game. Hard, real hard. I get mad. I get headaches, frustrated, 'cause I can't get the word, or sometimes I do get the word, but it didn't make sense to my head....She [his instructor] helps me on words I get stuck on, so I can keep going so the story will make sense. But I still concentrate too much on one word, trying to figure out what it is. In my mind, I forget what I read back there.

It's questionable whether Tom will persevere until he becomes an independent reader, in view of the frustration he often experiences, his lack of concentration and study habits, and the other demands in his life, including job demands.

Further, Tom is ambivalent toward the benefits that literacy will confer, despite his shame at being a nonreader. In this view, he told a little story about people who can read well but don't have much common sense. A friend of his who earned straight A's in school couldn't change his bike tire. Tom had to do it for him because Tom has common sense. He went on to tell me that I probably didn't have much common sense either; and when I said that I was pretty handy mechanically, he expressed disbelief. If Tom persists in the notion that book learning cancels out common sense, that the two are essentially mutually exclusive, he may not persist in the extremely hard work involved in becoming a reader.

Tom also does not believe that literacy is necessary for his job; he feels that he's pursuing this painful course for his own benefit. When asked to comment about the higher levels of skill demanded by changing technologies in the plant, he said that he stays away from any jobs that require anything like that, especially computers. When asked whether he would like to move into other jobs if he had the requisite skills, he responded not with desire but with the comment that he might have to do so at some point: the seniority system would force him into taking a job he would find very difficult because of his skill levels. Tom's main motivation is to make his money, not to move up in the ranks. His aspirations already have been met, in many ways.

Tom's supervisor already rated him highly as an employee. This supervisor added that Tom always had been self-motivated and a good, strong worker who made his quota of parts. He did say that since Tom has been in the program, he's found him more self-confident and more vocal about helping to solve problems on the new line. Tom, however, never needed supervision; he always "gave 110 percent" to the job. In that plant, in other words, Tom did high-quality work while totally illiterate.

Tom's perception of his literacy problems is quite accurate except for certain points such as believing that writing is mostly copying. He has particular insight about his reading abilities; he can diagnose his difficulty with comprehension of text as due largely to his lack of automatic word recognition skills. Tom also is now realistic about the amount of work he might require to become a more fluent reader. Even so, he is beginning to see himself as a reader with the potential to join the world of the literate.

Tom is also relatively accurate in his view that literacy skills have little effect on whether he can do his job well. In fact, he moved to another job designation, all-purpose operator, and on to a totally new line and manufacturing process—synchronous manufacturing—without knowing how to read, write, or do any mathematics beyond addition and subtraction of whole numbers. His perception of what the future holds, however, may be far less realistic, either his prospects of continuing at the plant or, if the plant is closed, for the possibility of a new job with another company. The automotive industry jobs surrounding Route 23 are continuing to disappear, although at least for now the union can provide more job security than most U.S. workers have.

Currently, however, Tom probably is a "successful" urban Appalachian male: a good provider for his family with a great deal of common sense, including intelligence and shrewdness. Yet his "swimming about in the mainstream," his probable biculturalism, somehow has caused him to feel a "blemish of personal character" without experiencing the "stigma of poverty."

This feeling of being blemished clearly led him to the learning center and into a literacy program. In the past, it also led him to several literacy agencies in the area in search of tutors to help him. Tom reported that none of those attempts succeeded, in part because the tutors gave up before Tom did so. One left on vacation, promising to call him back to resume instruction, but did not. The tutors' frustration is understandable because Tom represents a formidable challenge unless the instructor is relatively well trained. Further, he is not the type of person to return where he feels unwelcome.

Tom also showed little desire to learn any environmental print before entering the program at the plant. Although this behavior is not unusual among adult illiterates, Tom was intensely embarrassed at his inability to read the word *men* on men's room doors. Instead, he sent his wife to find out where the men's room was and to inform him. He also reported driving in great fear of getting lost if his wife was asleep in the car, because he couldn't read any signs. Nor would he wake up his wife, probably for fear of showing such rudimentary ignorance in front of his sons. His clear anguish over his lack of ability to read indicates deep dissatisfaction with himself as a nonreader. Even though his life was bounded by these fears, he did not try to solve problems by learning to recognize even a few words beyond the few necessary for driving as single, "unbreakable" units.

Although Tom is successful in many ways in his culture, this blemish has a powerfully corroding effect on his self-image. To put it another way, the pain of being a nonreader is worse than the pain of admitting and accepting that fact. Tom also is clearly in pain while learning to read; he finds it extremely difficult to deal with the language in the necessary metalinguistic manner. While learning to read, one must use language to think about that language-based activity. Also, one absolutely must look within words, into their components, and must coordinate sounds with letters on the decoding level. All of this activity must coordinate simultaneously with comprehending the text, with negotiating meaning between the reader and the text.

Such skills are complex and usually are acquired over a period of years while the reader is a child in school. Because this was not the case with Tom, he now is trying to weave all of these threads into whole cloth while fighting a lifetime of habitually avoiding reading. Meanwhile, he takes some solace from the realization that he has a good job, makes good money, and is respected by his peers and his supervisor. It remains to be seen, especially because the program at BodyWorks has ended and his instructor has departed, whether Tom will continue to struggle with such a difficult activity and will receive enough expert instruction to help him become "unblemished."

Harry

Harry is a 49-year-old urban Appalachian male with 24 years' seniority at BodyWorks. Currently, he is classified as a tool and die maker. He and his wife were married when they were both 17 and have three grown children. Their son, the youngest and the only male, has some of the same literacy problems as his father, which creates difficulties for him in college.

Harry did not graduate from high school; he earned a General Equivalency Diploma (GED) certificate. Although he can and does read a great deal for pleasure as well as for work, he would not write because of his attitude toward his spelling errors. He came to the learning center for help with his spelling so that he would feel comfortable writing.

Harry's feelings about his spelling abilities, which he believes are terrible, probably were instrumental in his dropping out of school. He said that during his junior year one of his teachers told him to go up to the blackboard to write something. Harry refused; the teacher insisted; Harry refused again. The teacher insisted again, and Harry took a swing at him. He was willing to fight rather than write on the blackboard. On that same day, he dropped out of his school in the Columbus public school system.

Nonetheless, Harry's literacy skills were developed highly enough to enable him to earn his GED and to serve two apprenticeships at BodyWorks. His first apprenticeship was in sheet metal; the second was in tool and die making. He served parts of his apprenticeship at a small local skills-oriented college, so he's even "darkened the doorstep" of an institution of higher education. In fact, Harry was interested in earning an engineering degree, as his son is doing now, but "couldn't"—actually wouldn't—take notes in class because of shame about his spelling. Because he couldn't memorize the material in the lectures and couldn't do well enough without notes, he did not pursue the degree.

Despite his work success, Harry was led to the center by these feelings surrounding his writing ability. When he was in the third grade, as he recalls, he was failed because of his spelling. He said he did well with his schoolwork in the year he repeated but received no effective help in spelling. At that time, he says, he began to memorize words and copy them verbatim for reports. That was the beginning of his feelings of inadequacy regarding spelling.

Now Harry feels he "can't spell at all." Although that is not the case—he can spell most of the words he writes—he focuses on the words he misspells to the exclusion of the others. He has become so extremely fearful of making spelling mistakes that he will not write anything that is not planned carefully in advance. For taking tests in school, for example, he worked out a series of possible answers ahead of time, memorizing the spelling of words he would use. Then he used his already-created answers when he took the tests. Harry also dropped out of typing class in high school when he learned, to his horror, that in typing he had to spell words "right now." He couldn't rely on his memory in that class. Thus, over the years, spontaneous writing has virtually disappeared from his literacy repertoire.

On his job as a tool and die maker at BodyWorks, Harry refuses to do any writing. This refusal is of long standing; 10 years ago he was asked to become a supervisor, a step above his current job. He refused because of his feelings about his "inadequate" spelling. He said he couldn't keep a journal, a necessity for the supervisory position, or write turnover reports, also absolutely necessary for that position.

Currently, Harry should leave notes for his counterpart on second shift telling what machines had what problems, what he did to fix them, what still needs to be done, and so on. Such turnover notes are standard practice for people in Harry's job. He refuses to do this, however, because of his shame about his spelling; he's terrified of misspelling a word. In fact, when his supervisor asked him to leave a turnover report, Harry told him that it wasn't part of his job description; if the supervisor insisted, he'd take it to the union grievance committee. Harry said he felt very bad about saying that. He wanted to cooperate, and usually he didn't do things like this because he really loves his job. Still, he couldn't face the thought of having to write something down for someone else to see. He can't leave an audio tape for the next shift because tapes are not part of the plant culture for turnovers. Workers don't leave tapes for one another; they leave notes. Any variation from this practice would invite comments, which Harry assiduously avoids. He, like Tom, is engaged in an elaborate coverup of his perceived lack of a literacy ability.

This scenario makes one wonder how many "uncooperative" workers are not really uncooperative but are fearful of displaying what they believe is ignorance in basic skills that most people have learned.

Harry also receives a fair amount of continued training on new machines and thus attends classes on repairing them. In that setting, he refuses to take any notes to aid his memory because the person sitting next to him might see his spelling errors. He also stated that he should keep notes, for himself and for others, on the repair record of specific machines. Harry has also been asked to create these logs but has refused to do so. Thus, his ability to do his job as well as he can is impaired because he will not do any writing.

Harry has tried to improve his spelling over the years, realizing that it is a barrier to performing his job as he would like to do it. He wrote the following description of the steps he's taken to learn to spell better:

I am a poor speller. I have tried many times to emprove my spelling but to no avil. A few of methods that I have tried are: Going over and over speller books, coursepondence [courses], privit tudor, home computer program called "Whole Brain Spelling," and reading a lot with the theory that if I see words many times eventually I would be able to spell. But nothing seems to work.

Spelling Diagnosis

The first step in diagnosing Harry's self-professed spelling problems was to ask him to describe them in his own words as specifically as he could. He felt he couldn't "visualize" words well enough. That is, he believes he relies mostly on sounding words out rather than having visual patterns stored in his memory. To back that contention, he said that at one point he had found himself a tutor in spelling. When working with her he had memorized the spellings of many words but had forgotten the spellings in a few months.

To illustrate, Harry showed how he had spelled *attentive* as *attenative*. He had tried to sound it out, breaking it into syllables. When he did so, he added a syllable that is not present in either the written word or in the spoken word. He said that he knew it wasn't right when he looked at it but couldn't diagnose what was wrong.

To help himself, Harry has purchased two electronic spellers of the type that is essentially a dictionary also programmed with common misspellings of words. A regular dictionary is often useless to him because he cannot begin the word correctly. Thus, he usually can't find the word. Dictionaries clearly are designed as reading rather than as writing aids. For example, Harry spelled *yeoman* as *yhoman*. Without knowing that the first syllable is spelled *yeo*, he could not find it in the dictionary, even if he knew something was wrong with his spelling. Another example is his spelling of *entrepreneur* as *antrapenor*. His spelling is very reasonable but of no help when he looks for the word under the A's in the dictionary.

Although Harry's electronic spellers are more helpful than a dictionary, they still present at least two problems. One is that he is ashamed of using it in front of most people and will not use it on the job. The other is that sometimes he misspells a word in an uncommon way. Those spellings are not programmed into the machine; thus, it will not produce any word at all. He is left where he was before—frustrated, ashamed, and forced to involve another human being in his problem.

Reading Diagnosis

Before addressing Harry's self-proclaimed spelling problem, I considered it important to obtain a sense of his reading ability: if he had word recognition difficulties in reading, a knowledge of those difficulties could help with the diagnosis of his spelling problems. It would allow for greater insight into "word handling" problems, both receptive (in regard to recognition while reading) and productive (in having to recall those words while spelling).

The first diagnostic instrument was the learning styles inventory used at the learning center. It revealed that Harry's favorite mode of learning was auditory-visual-kinesthetic ("hear-see-do"); preferences for learning from reading and for talking about what he knows ranked close behind. Not surprisingly, Harry eschewed writing as a way of learning, as well as learning in a group. Because reading as a mode of learning was rated quite high, it was even more important to gain some understanding of his reading abilities. Harry, however, also has what could be termed a "testing phobia": even when he was undergoing nontestlike, nonstandard-ized assessment procedures, he told me that his knees were shaking and his hands were sweating. In consequence, the interpretation of his results is difficult. They could be the result of his fear blocking his abilities, they could reflect his actual reading skills more accurately, or something between these two possibilities.

Therefore, I chose to ignore his scores on several of the instruments given to all employees in the learning center who could read well enough to take them. Tom, for example, was not assessed and diagnosed in any of these ways because he was a true nonreader, incapable of responding to the instruments. Harry could read, however. Yet his fears of even quasi-school situations were so pronounced that the results were likely to be skewed artificially toward the lower ends.

For the program, I devised a reading comprehension assessment instrument based on an analysis of meaning-bearing chains in the text (the Gap). The instrument also was based on text that was part of BodyWorks' manuals and training materials. Harry did rather well on that instrument; he said he had felt comfortable with it and that it made sense to him. Out of 12 blanks in the text, he replaced the missing word with the exact word five times, which is quite a good score. In five other instances, he used either a synonym of the missing word or a reasonable substitute in the same semantic field. On the basis of these results, it was clear that he understood the material.

To determine Harry's reading abilities even more clearly, I asked him to read aloud from work material he selected. Although reading aloud cannot reveal a great deal, it can demonstrate some important things about word recognition abilities, which in some ways are the "flip side" of spelling. Even this procedure terrified Harry; again, his knees shook and his palms sweated. He tackled it, however, and became more comfortable as he proceeded.

This procedure revealed that Harry has some sound-letter correspon-dence difficulties, including reversals. He read *G...A...S* for *AGS* and *adapt AM vision* for *Adept AIM version*. He also read *operator* for *operating* and *operation* for *operating*. In our discussion of the selection, it was clear that Harry understood what he had read. Although evidently he could read with meaning from a passage above the thirteenth-grade level, on the (FORCAST) readability scale, he has some word recognition problems that shed light on his spelling difficulties. For example, he does not always pay attention to vowels, where he makes most of his spelling errors. Also, he pays little attention to word structure, as when he read *operator* for *operating* (two different parts of speech). When inattentions to word structure and sounds are combined with his firm conviction that spelling is mostly memorization, we find that Harry did not have a pattern-seeking approach toward learning to spell.

This lack of pattern seeking shows clearly in his misspelled words. In some cases he spells a word the way he says it; and in other cases, he spells it as he thinks it should look. Thus, Harry's spelling is a complex combination of miscues from sound cues and visual cues, and a variable application of phoneme-grapheme correspondence rules. Over the years, he has taught himself some nonproductive spelling strategies.

For example, a given tense has a variety of graphemes, the so-called long vowel in English. This variety comes from the fact that in English we borrow words from other languages without anglicizing their spelling—for example, *parfait*, in which the spelling *ait* for *ay* is French. We also keep older phoneme-grapheme correspondence spellings, as in *knight* and *knife*. Harry selects one possible spelling for a vowel at one time and another at a different time. For example, he spelled *realized* as *realaized*. In some words, *ai* is the correct spelling for the tense vowel /ay/, but it is not correct in a word in which the tense vowel's grapheme is *i*/consonant/*e*, as is in *realize*. He essentially ignored the final *e*.

Harry spelled *hygiene* as *hiegen*. The first error, the *ie* for the *y*, is understandable. Yet because another vowel follows the consonant after the initial tense vowel, Harry should have known that the first vowel sound would not be spelled with a letter combination. The problem, then, is to determine which vowel letter is the correct one. Memory here is crucial because the word is borrowed from Hygia, the name of the ancient Greek goddess of health and cleanliness.

Harry misspelled the second tense vowel in *hygiene*, whose grapheme is *e*/consonant/*e*. Harry misspelled it with a single *e*. Again, that spelling breaks the common tense vowel grapheme patterns in English that require either a combination of two vowel letters together or the *vowel*/consonant/*e* combination.

When certain tense vowels occur at the ends of words, however, as in *sky*, they may be spelled with a single letter such as *y*. Harry also seems to have difficulty with this pattern and applies it inconsistently.

For example, he spelled *proximity* as *proxsimitie*. If we ignore for the moment the incorrect *s* inserted after the *x*, the *ie* was an incorrect choice for *y*, the usual pattern. When I pointed that out, he said something about words like *tie* and *die*. He is correct about that pattern, but it is a pattern for single-syllable words, not multisyllabic words. The most common spelling of the tense *i* at the end of a multisyllabic word is *y*, but Harry had not yet grasped that fact.

He also made a series of what could be called visually motivated omissions in spelling certain words. For example, he spelled *avail* as *avil*, *clutch* as *cluth*, and *wrench* as *wrenth*. For *avail*, one would normally expect the misspelling *aval* if the misspelling were sound motivated—that is, using the letter *a* to represent the tense vowel *a*. Harry used the *i* instead, almost as if he remembered that the word contained an *i* but forgot the other letter necessary for the grapheme *ai*. With *clutch* and *wrench*, the *th* grapheme does not make much sense in terms of sound. Again, it almost seems as if he remembered the *h* at the end, and knew that the graphemes required at least two letters, but couldn't get it right.

Possibly the clearest example of Harry's confusion with spelling patterns in American English is his spelling of *diamond,* which he spelled *diamound*. It appears as if he included the *o* by relying on his visual memory, but then said the word, heard the schwa / ∂ /, and added in the *u* to capture that "uh" sound we hear in /daym∂nd/.

Harry's spelling miscues are extremely complex; they combine elements of sound-based miscuing, visual pattern–based miscuing, and hybrid categories such as ignoring word boundaries to spell *in particular* as one word, *inpreticular*. The complexity stems in part from his many attempts to learn to spell better, which included assiduous reading of mass market books on how to improve spelling. None of the books he showed me are based on the actual patterns of American English traditional orthography, whether they are phonologically or morphologically based. Unless he works with the patterns, Harry stands virtually no chance of improving his spelling.

Harry as a Literate Worker

During his two months at the learning center, I diagnosed his spelling miscues from the writing he could bring himself to do. This work largely involved keeping logs on machine repairs, something he had wanted to do. Signs of his progress included a major change in attitude. He spent about $125 for a leather-bound organizer, which included note-taking space, and a Cross pen and pencil set, all of which he carried proudly on the factory floor and into the learning center. He began to make the logs in the organizer while on the floor at his station. One day he told me that an engineer, who was troubleshooting on one of the machines Harry was working on, noticed him making notes and joked, "Got to watch out for guys who take notes." By that remark, Harry was acknowledged as belonging to the ranks of writers, and he felt extremely proud. He also said he didn't feel self-conscious when taking notes at his bench, especially without using a dictionary, which he was finally able to put aside.

During the lessons, Harry and I worked on spelling patterns and on sharpening his ear to process pronunciation. Stress placement in words was especially important to Harry because stress is a major indicator of spelling patterns. He had never noticed this before and so could not possibly use it as a basis for cues. Sometimes he said something like, "I never had any idea that good spellers just didn't memorize the whole thing" or, "I never knew there were patterns like this."

In fact, Harry started to believe in patterns. Before this instruction, he said, he had memorized the letters in a word, "just like a telephone number." He had felt that the letters were in some random order with no rhyme or reason to them. "Now," he said, "I know it's there, a letter, because it has a certain function, like a long vowel sound or a short vowel sound." Harry also said, "Words now have a shape—not just a jumble of letters like they were before." He also was listening much more carefully for sounds in words.

We were not able to interview Harry's supervisor or talk with others in BodyWorks about changes they may have noticed in his work, because of his feelings of shame. Although these feelings diminished, they still prevented him from letting others know he was participating in the program. Therefore, we have only the anecdotal, self-reported information about what the engineer said to him about note taking, and about how he felt about taking notes when he attended various training sessions on machine repair. Evidently, change occurred, but it is also difficult to assess this change because Harry terminated instruction for the holiday break, and then the project ended.

Harry, like Tom, is a successful urban Appalachian male who holds a good job, has provided for his family, is an avid churchgoer, and has a variety of hobbies. Like Tom, however, he felt strongly the "blemish of person character"—in this case, his perceived inability to spell. This inability, according to Harry, blighted his life. While doing his best to find a way to improve his spelling over many years, he worked out a set of ways to hide this blemish from others, including his own children. As with Tom, it remains to be seen whether Harry will pursue more instruction to further "rid himself of his blemish." Unfortunately, it will be far more difficult for Harry to find such instruction than for Tom, because few people understand enough about the patterns of American English orthography to be able (1) to understand what Harry does when he misspells words, (2) to help him gain the necessary understanding of those patterns, and (3) to guide him through practice and to model a process of diagnosing misspelled words that he can internalize.

POLICY IMPLICATIONS

When members of a minority culture are adrift in the mainstream, and when that mainstream is a literate culture, they may feel blemished if they cannot read or write, or cannot do so at the levels they need in their lives or on their jobs. Literacy problems cannot be viewed as they are commonly seen by employers, politicians, popular writers, and even some educators, who bemoan the "lack of literacy skills" or the increasing, shameful levels of "adult illiteracy" in the United States. Most of this public outcry blames the victim or places such people squarely in the underclass, a new euphemism for the poor (Gans 1992). Tom, Harry, and Dick (the urban African-American) are not members of the underclass, nor are they victims in the usual sense of being unemployed, alienated individuals.

Tom and Harry are successful in many ways, both in urban Appalachian culture and in mainstream culture. They are law-abiding, tax-paying citizens. Yet from their own perspectives, as well as in the eyes of others, they are failures in one very important way: Tom could not read, and Harry would not write. They could not shrug off these failings, even though they tended to believe that book learning destroyed common sense. They were stigmatized in their own minds, and these stigmas led them to develop elaborate scripts for hiding their literacy problems. Finally, the stigmas also led them to the doors of the learning center, still in shame and with some secrecy, even though they were in their forties. Their other successes, considerable though they are, are not enough. For both men, literacy is a necessary accomplishment in the forms they are missing—reading for Tom and writing for Harry.

At this juncture, we can do little but wish them well, because they have few opportunities to continue expanding their literacy skills. This society provides almost no safety net for people who do not become accomplished enough in school to continue upgrading these skills on their own, as needed. Furthermore, most on-the-job training is intended for managers, not for skilled workers.

In thinking about policy implications growing out of the experiences of the Toms and Harrys, we first need to consider where literacy stigmatization begins. For many Appalachians it begins in school (Borman, Piazza, and Mueninghoff 1983; DeStefano 1990). In school the cultures may clash; there, according to Ogbu's (1988) oppositional framework, the desire to have common sense may well win out over the desire for book learning, and the decision to remain within the urban Appalachian community may lead to rejection of increases in a student's literacy repertoire.

Also, within many Columbus schools that have a significant urban Appalachian population, their values are hardly accommodated and their culture is hardly understood (DeStefano 1989). Many individuals in this group tend to fit the "image of poverty" (Precourt 1983) and also suffer the tribal stigma of race described by Goffman (Precourt 1983). Part of this stigma of race appears to be a lowering of expectations regarding the children's ability to become literate. Certainly the studies of Tom, Dick, and Harry in the first grade (DeStefano, Pepinsky and Sanders 1982) revealed that some patterns of Appalachian "failure" were established in the classroom as early as the first semester of the first grade, largely among those children whose families were on Aid to Dependent Children (ADC).

Tom and Harry did not come from homes on welfare. Their fathers were blue-collar workers, Tom's father at BodyWorks. Yet they, too, could have been branded with the tribal stigma of race, especially if they had displayed more dialectic features in their speech as young children. Their difficulties with literacy began very early in school, in the same pattern we see being established in schools with urban Appalachian populations in Cincinnati (Borman, Piazza, and Mueninghoff 1983). Tom, the nonreader at BodyWorks, said that his difficulty with reading had begun in the first grade. Harry's problems with spelling, or at least the problems he attached to spelling, became so serious that he was made to repeat the third grade.

Just as obviously, Tom and Harry remembered their experiences in school with distaste and not a little anger. Schooling as it existed then did not fit them, as it fails to fit all too many urban Appalachian children today. The continuing unequal impact on this particular group must be diagnosed carefully, and school policies and curricula must be adapted to meet these children's needs *and* gifts more effectively. One can only hope that book learning and common sense need not remain mutually exclusive and that the schools attended by urban Appalachian children can provide for the nurturing of both.

Another implication for educational policy involves the provision of opportunities for urban Appalachians after they drop out of school or graduate without the skills they may need to achieve their own goals, whether stable employment, further education, or providing more help to their children. Currently, almost no safety net is provided to them. The story repeats itself: they have difficulty in school for a variety of reasons (including hostility on the part of the school), they fail to learn, and then they are told essentially that they've had—and missed—their chance. It's the peacetime equivalent of Catch-22.

Both Tom and Harry sought specific education in literacy after they finished school. According to each of them, they could not find the type of instruction that would have enabled them to learn. Tutor after tutor disappeared from Tom's life; because of the difficulty of teaching an adult nonreader, this situation unfortunately is understandable. The typical community literacy programs depend on volunteers, usually with about eight hours of training; such programs tend to be most available to the Toms. These programs cannot deal with the complex set of literacy problems that the Toms usually have built up over the years; often, these problems include some degree of disability, which can challenge even a professional. Volunteers with no professional background in literacy simply cannot be expected to answer the needs of many urban Appalachians, either in providing effective literacy instruction or in understanding the culture and providing instruction that is more suited to them than were their school experiences.

Harry's many spelling books, his spelling "tudor," a software program for his home computer, and assiduous reading to familiarize his eye with words did not lead to better spelling. He has even fewer resources in the community than Tom, because adult spelling problems are understood far less than reading problems. The numbers of persons with serious spelling difficulties have not been estimated. Furthermore, few people know enough about the morphophonemic nature of traditional orthography to diagnose these individuals' problems. Yet their writing can be stalled or judged inadequate unless the spelling problems are resolved.

The workplace program instituted at BodyWorks, funded by the company and by the federal government, provided both Tom and Harry with their first real opportunity to participate in the specialized learning situation they needed to begin to overcome their difficulties. First, they came into contact with competent instructors. Second, the program was at their work site. Third, it afforded confidentiality during the initial phases when they seemed to need it most. (Relatively few employees demonstrated Tom's and Harry's need for virtual secrecy about coming to the learning center for instruction.) Undoubtedly, other program characteristics, such as a workplace orientation, also enabled them to experience the success they began to feel. Practicality was an advantage for Harry; this was one of his goals for writing. No workplace material could be used with Tom; it was too difficult for him while he was learning to read.

Community literacy programs that tend to concentrate on functional literacy (or survival literacy, as it is often called) need to be placed increasingly within an array of literacy services available to urban Appalachians. Often the workplace is the venue for "snagging" successful Appalachians such as Tom and Harry; at work, well-conceived programs can offer a level of instruction not available in many community programs. Adult basic education programs are another component of a successful array because they tend to concentrate on developing academic literacy abilities that usually lead to completion of the GED and to further schooling.

Thus, community policies must be worked out to establish the array of educational opportunities available in culturally relevant and acceptable ways, perhaps through neighborhood centers such as those in Cincinnati. Currently, Columbus has no such center for urban Appalachians, although an adult literacy umbrella organization is attempting to secure the funding to open one as a pilot in Franklinton, a portal neighborhood for urban Appalachians.

A final implication of this work with Tom and Harry concerns the workplace. Within labor-management relations, one must ask how much tension may be caused by some workers' inability to perform their jobs as well as they could or would wish because they lack certain basic literacy skills. Although an unhappy workplace is not based solely or even largely on workers' limited skills—poor management usually is a much bigger cause—American companies must provide nonthreatening, accessible educational opportunities for their employees. Certainly in Columbus, many economically successful urban Appalachians could be reached through the workplace and, through them, their homes and to their families.

The hopeful trip up Route 23 has brought economic success to some Appalachian migrants and to later generations. It has brought educational and other sorts of success to many as well. Even so, a "good job" does not necessarily secure the rights to a good education. Many urban Appalachians in Columbus are not stigmatized by the vicious stereotype of urban Appalachian poverty, often including the rusting refrigerator and the car up on blocks in the backyard, but are blemished by the lack of what they and others tend to regard as the proper level of literacy—as a set of personal characteristics. Neither stereotypes nor blemishes can explain much beyond people's feelings about themselves in relation to others, but they are indicative of victimization.

That which truly denies and victimizes is a complex interplay between cultures in contact, usually resulting in cultural clash. The casualties are suffered most frequently by those in subordinated cultures and often are revealed specifically in certain areas such as literacy. Reading and writing frequently are held hostage by the hostility among groups; the dominant society offers little hope of later recovery.

Therefore, "readin', writin', and Route 23" is more of a slogan or an exhortation than an indivisible trinity. The connection, however, can be strengthened and made more real so that the Toms and Harrys do not have to wander for years in the educational wilderness. Despite all of their successes, which were even more outstanding in the face of their literacy problems, they felt a hole in their beings: they were barred from written communication in a world full of writing. Their sense of incompleteness cannot be ignored, despite other people's definition of success. At the same time, their successes cannot be denigrated.

13

Social Change and Urban Appalachian Children: Youth at Risk

Kathryn M. Borman and Delores Stegelin

There was no doubt that these...[urban Appalachian] mothers cared about their sons and all the rest of the children in the family. But they were just trying to make ends meet and trying to hold themselves together, trying to meet the demands of the kids and it wasn't working. They seemed very overwhelmed.

Susan Murphy, Teacher
Cincinnati Public Schools

Change is a succession of differences in time in a persisting identity.

R. Nesbit

Nesbit (1972) defines the parameters of social change in terms of three elements: (1) differences (2) "in time" and (3) persisting identity. Change is not separable from the dimension of time. This chapter addresses the evolution of urban Appalachian children, youths, and their families through time as a part of social change. Social change affects adults directly in the frustrations, anxieties, and tensions it produces and in the opportunities and challenges it presents (Elkind 1979). The urban Appalachian mothers whose stories are described here are coping with their own immediate economic needs and problems. Their persistent struggles make it virtually impossible for them alone to provide the support that their children require to deal with their environments, especially school. Children and adolescents tend to be affected by social change indirectly through the adults who interact with them. Thus, children are influenced by social change primarily as it is manifested in adults' attitudes toward children and toward child rearing (Elkind 1979). In this chapter, we portray urban Appalachian children and youths who are overwhelmed largely because of the social changes occurring in their parents' lives.

The purpose of this chapter is to explore social change, particularly as related to health and education issues facing many low-income and marginalized Appalachian youths. The first section provides an overview of Appalachian migration history, including a focus on the stream of migrants who left eastern Kentucky for Cincinnati, a description of mountain people in Cincinnati, a view of urban Appalachian families and youths through the lens of literacy learning, and a description of work and health issues common to these mountain youths. We take data from two different studies: one probes work experiences and related values of Summer Youth Program participants, and the other examines literacy activities of Appalachian families. Data sources include participant observation as well as information gathered from personal interviews with urban Appalachian youths and their parents.

MOUNTAIN PEOPLE IN CINCINNATI:
SOCIAL CHANGE AND POVERTY

Data that profile 246 Summer Program participants present information on the conditions of young people who live in the Cincinnati neighborhood of Lower Price Hill (also see Chapter 11). This predominantly white community includes many families of third- and fourth-generation migrants from the Appalachian region. The youths include 21 teens who are either pregnant or mothers; the youngest is 14 years old. Household size ranges from one person ($N = 3$) to 9 individuals ($N = 3$); the modal household contains four family members ($N = 58$). The average annual family income reported by these youths is $7,788. Per capita income varies; the highest average per capita income ($12,312) is reported by those living in two-person households. The youths served by the Summer Program constitute approximately 50 percent of the adolescent population in the neighborhood and see themselves as both eager to better themselves and capable of doing so. These urban Appalachian youths may represent the least discouraged and therefore the least tough of the "tough cases" that characterize this group. Nonetheless, they speak eloquently for this population.

URBAN APPALACHIAN FAMILIES AND THEIR CHILDREN:
THROUGH THE LENS OF LITERACY

Urban Appalachian families form tight units that become the centers for home learning and for cultural rites and passages. Literacy is an important indicator of both functions, creating skills and tools for economic advancement and advantage in the marketplace (Courts, 1991). By examining literacy, we can learn more about the intricate relationship between the Appalachian family and home, the school, and the community. From a research project developed and conducted by the Center for Research on Literacy and Schooling at the University of Cincinnati, we collected data on Appalachian families. The children of these families were the subjects of literacy research in their neighborhood school classrooms. We also visited their homes to more clearly understand the critical links existing among children, homes, communities, and schools, particularly as related to literacy development.

Previous studies demonstrated the importance of links between children's school achievements and family behaviors, family composition, and socioeconomic status. Data are lacking, however, for explaining the patterned variations in the interrelationships of these variables. One goal of the literacy research project was to identify and compare links between family and school that predicted Appalachian children's literacy learning success in school.

Literacy Linkages between Family and School

Numerous researchers have identified family activities that enhance literacy development in young children. Heath (1983) and Snow and Ninio (1986) identified such activities as storybook reading, experimenting with writing, and the use of print as providing young children with school-related knowledge that prepared them for the transition from home to formal education. Dahl, Purcell-Gates, and McIntyre (1989) found that inner-city children with knowledge of written language were more successful than others at learning to read and write in a traditional public school kindergarten classroom. In a study of low-income Latino families, Reese et al. (1989) concluded that the "impact of parents' educational experiences on children is mediated through particular activity settings, such as the use of literacy behaviors at home, the viewing of incipient child literacy attempts in a positive and encouraging light, and the scaffolding of children's learning experiences" (p. 20).

Family Literacy Activities

In order to assess the literacy activities of the urban Appalachian families, we developed a literacy scale. This scale took into account such variables as storybook reading, experimenting with writing, and the use of print activities, all of which help prepare children for success in school. As indicators of family literacy activity, we also included the parents' reading and writing experiences and the literacy environment of the household, including the availability of printed matter. We found moderate and even strong relationships among literacy activities and the variables of socioeconomic status and family educational practices and experience, whereas the relationships between family literacy scores and school success were more limited.

Our analyses show that in urban Appalachian families, family practices (literacy activities, approaches to discipline, and school participation) are highly interrelated. Urban Appalachian families who have more exposure to family literacy experiences also are more authoritative (rather than authoritarian) in their disciplinary practices and participate more frequently in their child's school activities. As we noted above, however, the relationship between these practices and students' achievement is weak. Family literacy has a strong association with parents' school participation and a rather weak association with authoritative parenting. None of the other family variables, however, have any predictive power with respect to school-based outcomes such as teacher-assigned reading grades or students' reading scores as measured by the California Achievement Test. Therefore, this study reveals the ability of the close-knit Appalachian family to promote parents' school participation as well as to provide the hub for literacy learning. One implication that we derived from this study is the clear need for more home-based and family-centered interventions in the form of parent-child literacy activities, as well as the need to make teachers aware of the nature of home-based family literacy activities.

WORK, HEALTH, AND SCHOOL DYSFUNCTION: ELEMENTS OF SOCIAL CHANGE IN JOBS AND WORK

Once they arrived in the cities, Appalachian migrants followed a well-documented and strategic pattern of settlement in port-of-entry neighborhoods. In Cincinnati, for example, migrants relied on established networks of kin to provide entry to the workplace. This livelihood strategy is consistent with patterns of cooperation and interdependence characteristic of mountaineers. Migrant workers recruited kin to jobs in the city during the manufacturing boom years; this process, according to some estimates, resulted in the employment of as many as 70 percent of Kentucky-born workers in many Cincinnati plants. The major settlement patterns in Cincinnati occurred in neighborhoods such as Lower Price Hill and Over-the-Rhine. These areas were adjacent to the highly industrialized Mill Creek Valley, where jobs were literally within walking distance. From the 1940s into the 1970s, the Appalachians worked in factories and small sheet metal and machine tool shops at jobs that generally required little or no experience or training.

In the 1980s and 1990s, urban Appalachian youths have remained economically marginalized. Youths from low-income families often avoid more challenging opportunities outside their neighborhoods because such jobs disrupt important social networks of exchange among kin and peers. Such opportunities often create cultural conflicts that cannot be resolved easily. Because youths lack experience in negotiating such conflicts, employers view them as expendable workers. Lacking adequate mentors, role models, and sponsors, the youths may continue to drift, keeping afloat with a series of odd jobs and exchange strategies. During the 1980s, unskilled work in manufacturing jobs was scaled back because of automation and the general decline of manufacturing jobs in an increasingly service-based national economy. Thus, many third- and fourth-generation urban Appalachian families remain isolated and out of work.

Youths living in urban Appalachian enclaves are particularly vulnerable; they attend schools that maintain patterns of socioeconomic segregation. Although socioeconomic status as defined by parents' income and education is generally a strong predictor of alienation from school (reflected in the dropout rate), the relationship is by no means perfect. In Cincinnati, for example, the dropout rates of some urban Appalachian neighborhoods are even higher than would be suggested by their socioeconomic ranking relative to other city neighborhoods. In one such case, according to the 1980 census data, a relatively high-ranking neighborhood (17th of 44) in socioeconomic status had the eighth-highest dropout rate in the city.

Discrimination against urban Appalachians persists in the current job market. In cities such as Detroit, Chicago, Cleveland, Columbus, and Cincinnati, in which large urban Appalachian populations live alongside established white groups, urban Appalachians without the benefit of middle-class origins and a college education do not acquire jobs and income equal to those of other whites. According to a political and economic analysis of job mobility and labor market conditions (Philliber 1981a), neither cultural differences nor migrant status, alone or in combination, account for this outcome. Rather, Appalachians are excluded in order to reduce the competition for jobs "reserved" for native non-Appalachian whites.

Analysts have concluded that the labor market is actually segmented. One segment is the primary or institutionalized labor market, which contains well-paying jobs, a career ladder internal to the work organization, and an evaluation of performance on the job based on clear criteria. In contrast, positions in the secondary labor market have few advantages: jobs pay poorly; hours are irregular and/or part-time; there is little or no opportunity for advancement; and although evaluation might appear to be objective because of the employer's use of rating sheets, it is influenced heavily by the informal social relations between employer and employee in the work setting (M. Miller 1981).

The promise of stable, well-paying employment remains elusive for urban Appalachian youths whose repertoire of skills and behaviors places them at odds with employers' biases toward persons with a more "appropriate" demeanor. Employers want docile, "responsible" workers who are without strong obligations to kin, who have none of the problems associated with young families of their own, and whose approach to life is less spontaneous and less engaged than that of many urban Appalachian and black youths. In their survey of youths in Baltimore, Providence, Cincinnati, and Detroit, McCoy and McCoy (1987) determined that of those who were of school age but not in school, 49.2 percent were Appalachian, 46 percent were other ethnics (including Hispanic and Polish), and 4.7 percent were black. For the most part, Appalachians and other white ethnics simply had dropped out of school. In contrast, a large minority (25%) of blacks had disrupted educational careers because of criminal convictions, resulting in their incarceration and withdrawal from school (McCoy and McCoy 1987).

Health-Related Issues for Appalachian Youths

Health-related issues for children are increasingly important in the United States, principally as a result of economic hardships confronting children and their families. Children under age four now make up the greatest segment of the poverty population in our country (Children's Defense Fund 1990); one of every four preschoolers in the United States lives in poverty. With the continuing recession, families who once were financially secure are now facing hardship. It is estimated, for example, that 250,000 children in the United States are homeless. Homelessness is increasingly a threat to formerly middle-income families. In addition, AIDS (Acquired Immune Deficiency Syndrome) is increasing in the preschool population, as is the population of children affected by their parents' cocaine and crack use. Contemporary U.S. society has begun to address school learning and behavioral difficulties in places such as New York City and Chicago, where some of the first so-called crack babies now are of school age. Teachers of these children are reporting a range of learning problems and failures: these children have difficulty in learning to spell their names, in attending to the teacher as a story is read, and in following routines such as lining up at the classroom door. It is not yet clear to what extent "crack children" will place an increased burden on the schools that receive them. Nor is it clear whether cities other than New York, Chicago, and Los Angeles will have many of these and other children whose severe learning and behavioral disorders are associated with extreme maternal substance abuse.

Although urban Appalachian children and youths in Cincinnati may not suffer the effects of severe maternal drug abuse and early addiction, there is little question that health issues, combined with community social and economic decline (as suggested above), contribute to early school dysfunction and later to dropping out of school. A five-year study of hospital admissions for children from infancy to age 11 revealed the links among neighborhood residency, pollution, other health hazards, and patterns of diagnosis (see Chapter 7; Lower Price Hill Task Force 1990).

It is difficult to know the effects of children's health-related problems on school functioning. Yet as school systems become oriented increasingly to evaluating students' performance from a point early in their careers, it is likely that health-related issues will come increasingly to play an explicit rather than a tacit role in how students are tested, evaluated, and classified. Indeed, in Cincinnati Public Schools today, children from low-income urban Appalachian neighborhoods have higher rates of identifiable learning problems than do children from the city at large. Achievement scores as measured by the California Achievement Test have declined overall over the past five years for students in grades 1 through 6, but the decline among urban Appalachian children is two to three times greater for the district as a whole (Lower Price Hill Task Force 1990).

Among older urban Appalachian children and youths, other health-related issues predispose them to be at risk for school dysfunction leading to school leaving. Pregnancy and early parenthood are prominent among these issues.

Among the 246 Summer Youth Program participants aged 14 to 21, 12 percent were either pregnant or parents. None of these individuals, however, were among the young men and women we interviewed during the summer of 1991. These young women were particularly disdainful of their pregnant and parenting peers and also expressed a lack of interest in traditional female interests. One of them remarked:

Where I live there's [lots of guys] and about four or five girls....Some of them don't come out at all because they're scared [of neighborhood fights]. They aren't allowed out, and so I usually hang with all the guys.

Another young woman, who was clearly a leader among these girls, clarified her friend's statement:

What she's trying to say is that you can do more with the guys...[general snickering] not sexwise...but you can hang out more with them and do what they do. Girls just want to fix their hair and stuff, but guys...want to get down and party, and play football.

Perhaps because of their participation in the Summer Program, these young women had clear ideas about their future work plans and maintained a firm resolve to avoid early pregnancy and motherhood. All wanted to pursue occupations that required at least two years of college. In contrast, young women whose interests are more traditionally feminine may be more likely to view pregnancy as attractive, particularly when the neighborhood offers few other options.

Among young men the greatest health risks are linked to the violence that visits their neighborhood in the forays by gangs of more affluent whites from "the hill." Program participants spoke of two or three age-mates from the neighborhood who had been "wasted" in gang-related activity, although they vigorously denied the presence of gangs from the neighborhood.

In sum, work- and health-related issues may predispose young urban Appalachian children to perform less well in school. School-related factors also inhibit their success, however. Both the structure of the schooling and the relationship of the school to the broader community must be considered in any analysis of children's school-related difficulties.

COMMUNITY LIFE AND EDUCATIONAL ISSUES

In describing the dilemmas of community life for residents of Cincinnati's urban Appalachian neighborhoods and particularly for children and their families, we now examine the circumstances of urban Appalachian children, youths, and their families. First we discuss how young children negotiate neighborhood life. Next we consider how older urban Appalachian youths survive on the streets and how they and their families manage the "welfare game." These accounts have implications both for educational policy and for social service policies in general.

Growing Up as an Urban Appalachian:
Negotiating the Neighborhood in the Elementary School Years

Life in predominantly urban Appalachian neighborhoods varies according to the economic prosperity enjoyed by neighborhood residents. In Cincinnati neighborhoods such as Over-the-Rhine, Lower Price Hill, and the East End, households face severe economic constraints that limit the resources available for use on the children's behalf.

The residents of Lower Price Hill have settled in the neighborhood over a period of 25 to 30 years, migrating in a clearly identifiable, coherent, consistent stream from eastern Kentucky coalfields. Their migration pattern is similar to that of nearly all urban Appalachian communities. Close kin tended to move to the same location in the city; they provided shelter, support, and access to jobs for relatives who arrived later. In a group of 24 parents living in Lower Price Hill, 1 named 30 relatives living in the neighborhood (Borman, Piazza, and Mueninghoff 1983). Only 1 respondent had no relatives living nearby; most had 7 or more. As a result of these settlement patterns and subsequent sustained interactions, children in Lower Price Hill grow up in a context of familial ties.

The neighborhood's topography contributes to the close integration and the sense of isolation from the rest of the city. Observers regularly characterize the neighborhood as an urban "holler." Geography makes Lower Price Hill an enclave community because a steep, unpopulated hill encloses it to the north; highways, major thoroughfares, and a viaduct spanning the Mill Creek Valley surround it on other sides. Because of these boundaries, children in Lower Price Hill develop a clear sense of their community. When a group of 10 children (ages 7 to 14) and their parents were asked to make an outline of their neighborhood on a city street map, the children responded by drawing a space more circumscribed than that drawn by their parents. All of the children agreed upon a core area that included frequently used social spaces such as the elementary school and the surrounding yard, the Bible Center, a social service agency housing a community council meeting room, the locally controlled community school, and other offices accessible to the neighborhood.

Borman, Piazza, and Mueninghoff (1983) investigated children's use of neighborhood social services to gain an understanding of their involvement in neighborhood social life during the summer months when they were not in school. Three basic assumptions guided this research. First, children who spent recreational time outside their homes were viewed as gaining important knowledge about patterns of social participation in community activities. Among adults, such involvement apparently generates satisfaction with one's role in the community. A second assumption was that children who were active participants in neighborhood life were building strongly positive feelings about their neighborhood. A third assumption, following from our knowledge of settlement patterns, was that kin groups and informal friendship networks were important in determining knowledge and use of community resources by neighborhood children and youths. Therefore, the children's involvement in neighborhood life not only would reflect their perceptions of benefits from such involvement but also would depend strongly on their integration into a network of neighborhood friendships and family relationships.

Several findings in this study bear comment. First, the children have a working knowledge of their neighborhood and its resources, as shown by their responses to the boundary-drawing task mentioned above. Second, by age 7, the children develop generally positive and strong emotions about their neighborhood. In response to the question "If you had to explain to someone where you lived, what would you say?" the youngest respondent replied, "I live over there [pointing across the street] where my cousins live." A slightly older child (age 8) responded, "Here, the schoolyard by Oyler School, my house, and my friends.' " A 12-year-old said, "To me it's the only community I've ever lived in. It's my life."

Finally, children learn of ongoing activities in the neighborhood by word of mouth. Many informal activities, street games, and the like, are undertaken by children who live in the same buildings and gather spontaneously after lunch or in the evenings on street corners or playgrounds. Other activities, such as events at the Bible Center, are more regularized because they are scheduled at specific times. A 13-year-old newcomer to the neighborhood was representative in naming the Bible Center (open weekdays from 10:00 A.M. to 2:00 P.M.) as the primary social center for children: "I met a kid down the street who brought me up here [to the Center]. So far I've been here two weeks—I like to play Ping-Pong."

The attractiveness of the Bible Center was based on two features, both important in understanding political socialization in the neighborhood. First, the supervisor was a local resident, the 18-year-old daughter of a prominent, civically active neighborhood family who provided activities appealing to children of many ages. Although the local social service agency paid her salary, her family had donated the pool table and Ping-Pong equipment used by older children. Art supplies were available for the younger children's projects. Second, because the facility was located in the geographical center of the neighborhood, it served as a convenient place to meet other children.

In summary, children in the enclave investigated here are informed by their working knowledge of local geography and by word-of-mouth communication, and they make use of neighborhood resources. They favor formally provided social services; these are most popular when supervision is locally based. These findings have direct application to policies aimed at eliminating traditional patterns of school organization that are bureaucratic and centralized rather than site based.

Growing Up as an Urban Appalachian: "Handling It Myself" in Adolescence

In extremely dysfunctional families, ambivalence about schooling is reduced to indifference simply because the family's immediate needs are so overwhelming. Susan Murphy, the Cincinnati Public School teacher whose statement about urban Appalachian mothers and their sons began this chapter, observed that the transition from the interdependence of family members that characterizes life in rural Appalachia has not necessarily been made in the urban Appalachian context.

Susan described the mothers of her fourth- and fifth-grade students, boys who were having difficulty in school and who had been assigned to her special education class. This class was designed for students with severe behavioral disorders.

All of these women, I remember very vividly and exactly what they looked like. They were real open and, like their sons, were easy to get close to, but [they were] overwhelmed. [They were]...deeply caring, but [they] did not know what to do for the kids. They had no control...could not make them come in at night...could not make them go to bed....could not make them get up and come to school. The sons were more or less running their own show. The mothers had lost control, which is a big problem when one of the kids gets in trouble with the law. [The mothers] could parent the younger ones, but once...[their sons] grew up, what could...[the mothers] do with somebody they considered to be on the same level?

Susan Murphy's observations on strained family networks and the difficulties facing young mothers in the city underscore the issues that face both the young mother and the child for whom inadequacy of family resources creates an uncertain figure. Earlier we pointed out that urban Appalachians constitute the largest group of students (in proportion to their numbers) who leave school in Cincinnati before graduation. Among young women, as mentioned previously, school leaving is most often associated with pregnancy.

Street Life and Welfare

For boys and young men, school leaving is connected with what one survivor of that lifestyle calls "living on the streets" or "handling it myself." Larry Redden, who grew up on the streets and survived to return as a youth worker, vividly describes his early experience. He contrasts his opportunities with the limited supports available to youths today and discusses the young people's activities with a particular emphasis on street culture and behavior. Larry, a first-generation urban Appalachian, recalls that his move to the streets originated with his family's need to play the welfare game. His family's experiences are not atypical; they illustrate several important points, especially the strategies, the life stresses, and the resilience of these individuals.

Growing up with family that came from the eastern part of Kentucky and the West Virginia area, my first house was approximately at 328 Third Street down in the bottoms. The bottoms were the houses on stilts so the flood waters wouldn't get in.

When I was born, my mother was on welfare, which caused a problem. She had my older sister with her, but at that point in time, being on welfare, you weren't supposed to have a man in your life....No kind of man was supposed to be even around, or else you could get kicked off welfare. That created a problem for my mother when she was pregnant because once she went to the hospital, she would have been cut off welfare because of being with a man.....That was certainly proof that she had been with a man within the last nine months.

When she went to the hospital, she used a fictitious name. She took her middle name, took my father's name, and cut off the last letters and added others, which made her be Louise Redding. My father did the same, so when I was born, I was born as Larry James Redding instead of Redden. My mother said other people did that and that she got the idea from a friend of hers.

Winning the welfare game required the kind of resourcefulness that prompted Larry's mother to give Larry a fictitious surname at birth. To stay afloat economically as Larry grew up, the family had to relocate frequently to more affordable housing. As a result of these relocations, Larry changed schools frequently. As he points out in the narrative below, he had attended five different elementary schools, yet he managed to earn high grades.

From the bottoms, we moved to Riverside, which was in a house that was really close to the [Ohio] River, and every year we used to be flooded out. My mother was still living on welfare. Then we moved into Laurel Homes because in a sense it was like subsidized housing back in the early fifties. I went to Washburn School. We moved to Vine Street, which was basically Over-the-Rhine, and from about age 6, that was where I grew up. That's the beginning—my kind of life living on welfare. Between the ages of 6 and 7 I went to five different schools. The remarkable thing is that I did very well. I was a straight-A student and very rarely ever got a B. When I transferred to junior high, I started failing. That was at the same time when I started living on my own. I was almost 12, and I was out on the streets on my own. The reason for that was that we were sitting in the house on Vine Street and a welfare worker came in without knocking. She just opened the door, and we had a television, a little Philco TV that my uncle had given us because we didn't have a radio or TV or anything in the house. At that point in time, you weren't allowed to have what they called "luxuries" in the house, or you would be thrown off welfare.

To play the welfare game, families must adapt to a survival that is highly stressful from both folk and bureaucratic perspectives. The strains become wrenching when government policies force families to break apart, as in Larry's case.

CONCLUSION

As a social worker serving the urban Appalachian community, Larry Redden sees both the possibilities and the constraints inherent in current social service policies: "In our city today, we've got maybe a thousand...[social service] agencies and organizations in the network, and the targeted population is the black community." This situation is far different from Larry's experience when he was growing up: "Then it seemed like everyone fell short of having that sort of service. There weren't any services for anyone then, so we made do with what we had. Today society offers programs, but it puts constraints on them as to who will be eligible." Federally funded programs do not target urban Appalachians, who generally are not recognized as a minority group according to federal guidelines.

Although individual characteristics such as early pregnancy, employment discrimination, and health-related issues may contribute to early school leaving, a clear relationship also exists between school leaving, truancy, and failure, and such school-related features as high rates of student suspension, low overall reading achievement, and high rates of absenteeism. Even though urban Appalachian children may leave school, they regard education and learning as very important. They are concerned about racial equality and opportunities for both blacks and whites. Moreover, families value the skills learned in school and view them as essential both for performing certain tasks and for finding a job as an adult.

Stegelin (1992) reviews the policy shifts needed for the 1990s and cites the critical at-risk child population, which is escalating in the United States. More specifically, in considering policy shifts and needed reforms appropriate for urban Appalachian youths and their families, we offer suggestions derived from conversations with people such as Larry Redden. These individuals are based in the community and have survived by beating the odds and skillfully negotiating the system. Two major problems persist in current service delivery: (1) the services made available to the community by bureaucracies overlap and are almost impossible to negotiate, and (2) little effort is made to target problems peculiar to urban Appalachians or to recognize them as a group eligible for services.

14

Appalachians in Cities:
Issues and Challenges for Research
Rhoda H. Halperin

In this concluding chapter, I outline a set of general issues and challenges for research among working-class Appalachians in cities. By *cities*, I mean contexts, both geographical and cultural, that are defined officially as urban but that have many hidden features not usually associated with urban areas. The issues discussed here are wide-ranging and serious from scholarly and scientific as well as from community (neighborhood) and policy perspectives. I shall be painting with a very broad, somewhat unconventional, and perhaps controversial brush; the questions I pose and the positions I take here will not necessarily be popular or even familiar in the academy; neither will they necessarily echo the positions taken by advocacy organizations.

If a set of assumptions must be acknowledged (and indeed no social scientist conducts research without assumptions), two are most important: first, the approach taken here is anthropological in the most classic sense. The aims are to understand how Appalachian people live and work in cities, to analyze the patterns and variations in beliefs and behaviors, and to uncover the origins of these patterns and variations. This approach includes, in more current anthropological parlance, listening to multiple voices—to many, often very dissonant, discourses—and trying, at the same time, to keep the channels of communication open. Second, in order to work as a researcher, it is necessary to adopt the position of an advocate in the most proactive sense of the term. At the same time, advocacy for certain community issues must not be allowed to stand in the way of the research process. In more mundane terms, advocates cannot risk alienating parts of the community.

Although this chapter does not focus on any particular Appalachian community, it is written from the perspective of a researcher/advocate with long-term ethnographic experience in both rural and urban

Appalachian communities. These experiences have taught me that there is no such thing as a neutral stance in Appalachian communities. That is, in order to work effectively as a researcher, one must adopt the position of an advocate at least to the degree that the good of the community (however *good* and *the community* are defined) underlies the data collection process. Given the difficulties of building consensus and the omnipresence of political factions at the local level, adopting an advocacy position involves a constant and delicate balancing act. Nonetheless, the opposite is impossible: to try to adopt a neutral stance is to distance oneself to the point of rejection or, at best, to lose access to critical data that can be used by the communities for a variety of purposes, including increased empowerment and the recognition of the strengths of grass-roots leadership and community itself. Throughout this chapter, although I am careful to maintain strict confidentiality and therefore use only fictitious names for people and places, I describe specific examples of people and places to illustrate the general points.

Certain hard questions are necessary to ask if we are to conduct high-quality research and if this research is to respect and enhance the diversity, energy, and richness of Appalachian people in cities. Giving up power and titles, fighting the ethnocentrism of even the most well-intentioned do-gooders and city officials, and being a diplomat without selling out to the dominant institutions must all be done in cooperation with community leaders.

In urban contexts, defining (analytically) and identifying (empirically) Appalachian people are difficult because Appalachians reside among non-Appalachians and because people who are third-, fourth-, or fifth-generation urban dwellers may or may not wish to identify themselves with any particular (Appalachian) geographical area. I suggest a three-pronged approach to identifying Appalachians in cities, based on geographical, cultural, and social structural factors.

The three-pronged approach consists of geographical, cultural, and social structural factors. Geography refers to place of origin; culture refers to rural experience; and social structural factors refer to the importance of the extended family, especially intergenerational ties. Together these three factors create the threads of Appalachian ethnicity and identity. They allow us to understand Appalachians of European origin as well as Appalachians of African-American origins in the rural South. They also allow us to understand the interactions between Appalachians in cities and Appalachians in rural areas, including the mountains of Kentucky, West Virginia, and Tennessee.

The questions researchers formulate must be rethought with sensitivity to community reactions to data collection and presentation:

What kinds of data should be collected? What circumstances—local, regional, and national—set the agendas for data collection and for advocacy? What are the roles of community leaders and community institutions in setting research agendas and in organizing and disseminating information about communities? The timing of data collection and dissemination is critical here. What are our units of data collection and analysis—individuals, families, households, communities, regions? The relationships between researchers and urban institutions ranging across universities, advocacy organizations, and social service agencies raise further questions about who is to use the data and for what purposes.

As an anthropologist, my own predispositions for in-depth ethnography (a people-centered, personal approach that is empathic and also analytical in its awareness of the larger forces impinging daily on people's lives) far outweigh the important but nonetheless more impersonal "number-crunching" approach to social science research. For Appalachians in cities, many of whom must struggle daily to maintain their close family and neighborhood relationships in the face of impersonal urban institutions, a research methodology that supports and reinforces personal, face-to-face relationships is certainly worth considering, even though ethnography is highly labor-intensive and thus expensive. Ethnographers should collect quantitative data, but those data must be collected and analyzed in specific social, cultural, and historical contexts that are necessary to understand qualitatively in order to make sense.

An anthropological approach also derives necessarily from a comparative, cross-cultural perspective that views Appalachian people in cities as sharing many of the same experiences as rural-urban migrants in cities around the world. For example, Appalachian children in cities may have at least as much in common with those children whose voices Oscar Lewis (1961) recorded from a barrio in Mexico City, as with rural Appalachian children in, say, the hills of Kentucky. The reasons for these commonalities are complex: they can be explained, however, at least in part, by the fact that Appalachian people in cities and barrio dwellers in urban Mexico both originate in rural (peasant) communities.

In such communities, extended families are the keystones of social organization, and intergenerational ties (especially between children and their grandparents but also between mothers and daughters and fathers and sons) are the most important social relationships. These ties outweigh occupational statuses; responsibilities to members of extended families outweigh obligations in school or on the job.

FINDING APPALACHIANS IN CITIES:
ETHNICITY, GEOGRAPHY, OR BOTH

Many Appalachian people who currently live in cities such as Cincinnati have been urban residents for three to five generations. If one phrases the question "Where are your people from?" a variety of responses will be forthcoming: European countries such as Ireland, Scotland, England, France, and Germany constitute one set of responses. Appalachian states such as Kentucky, West Virginia, and Tennessee are another set. In many instances, a part of the kin network came directly from Europe to the city; in other instances, some or all of the kin network came initially to a rural part of the Appalachian region. In almost all cases, however, people move back and forth between country and city. The movement of people refers not to residential instability but to people, especially children, visiting frequently on weekends and spending time with relatives on holidays.

If one asks a fifth-generation urban dweller in a so-called Appalachian community whether he or she is Appalachian, the answer, in most working-class communities, will be negative. The best way to identify Appalachian origins is not by asking people about themselves but by asking about their ancestry. Discussions of ancestry will reveal not only geographical origins but also key features of family and community organization. Geographical origins include the rural South; the mountains in the Appalachian region; and the rural areas of states, many of them nonmountainous, that are included in the Appalachian region. Appalachians originate from rural areas (in the United States and in Europe) in which the extended family is the most important unit of social organization.

URBAN AND *APPALACHIAN*: A CONTRADICTION IN TERMS?

The term *urban Appalachian* is a problematic, if not a contradictory, term. The term is difficult for several reasons. First, I can think of no other migrant population to whom the term *urban* has been attached. We do not write of urban Vietnamese, urban Hispanics or Latinos, urban Italians, or urban Chinese. Yet many migrated from rural settings that are very similar to those from which so-called urban Appalachians came. Second, the term is not recognized by "the folk" for whom it was meant. In fact, it is often rejected by people whose families originated in rural Kentucky, West Virginia, or Tennessee. Although the causes for rejection are complex, and although many people reject the term

Appalachian (rural or urban) because they equate it with *hillbilly, ridge-runner,* or some other stereotype (McCoy and Watkins 1981), it is also true that there is a certain artificial quality to the term *Appalachian* in that it is not indigenous; it is imposed from outside.

For analytical purposes, if we oppose the terms *urban* and *Appalachian,* we may learn more about Appalachians in cities than if we lump them together (see Friedl 1983). To consider these terms together is, in some important ways, to equate "urban" with "Appalachian" or to assume that Appalachians share or accept features of urban life that they, in fact, resist vehemently.

Working-class and poor Appalachian people in cities, first and foremost, are people who feel most comfortable in "the country" or in small-scale, face-to-face social settings; who invent and re-create such settings in the midst of cities; and who give priority to family, kin, and neighborhood obligations even when these conflict with obligations to jobs, schooling, and other tasks defined by the urban power structure as important. I am not saying that Appalachian people are attached to the land; I am saying that attachments to place and to family, which originated in rural areas of the United States and are common in all rural agrarian societies in nation-states, can be seen among Appalachians in cities, albeit in different forms. In fact, extended families are important to the very survival of working-class people in cities (Borman, Piazza, and Mueninghoff 1983; Halperin 1990).

On many fronts, working-class Appalachians are actively involved in resisting city ways. Priorities for sharing one's resources, however meager, and priorities that place responsibilities for kin and neighbors above personal needs and wants, result in a resistance to upward mobility. Personal relationships take precedence over bureaucratic dealings and skills. In some instances, mere contact with a bureaucracy such as city government—even going to city hall and feeling comfortable there—might be interpreted by one's fellow community members as "working for the city," that is, selling out the community. While often Appalachian resistance is regarded negatively by the keepers of urban institutions—including teachers and city officials (and the clerks who work for these officials)—much of their resistance must be regarded positively if Appalachian identity and heritage are to be respected and maintained.

In a poignant passage from *The Dollmaker* (1954), her classic story of rural-urban migration, Harriet Arnow describes one kind of resistance to urban institutions. The voice of Gertie, the main character, who, upon having a conference with her son's teacher over his poor grade in conduct, laments the following:

"I see no point in carrying this discussion further. He will have to adjust."

"Adjust?" Gertie strode ahead, turned and looked at the woman.

"Yes," Mrs. Whittle said, walking past her. "That is the most important thing, to learn to live with others, to get along, to adapt one's self to one's surroundings."

"You teach them that here?" Gertie asked in a low voice, looking about the dark, ugly hall.

"Of course. It is for children—especially children like yours—the most important thing—to learn to adjust."

"You mean," Gertie asked—she was pulling her knuckle joints now—"that you're a teachen my youngens so's that, no matter what comes, they—they can live with it?"

Mrs. Whittle nodded. "Of course."

Gertie cracked a knuckle joint. "You mean that when they're through here, they could—if they went to Germany—start gitten along with Hitler, er if they went to—Russia, they'd git along there, they'd act like the Russians and be—"

Mrs. Daly's word was slow in coming—"communists—an if they went to Rome they'd start worshipen the Pope?"

"How dare you?" Mrs. Whittle was shrill. "How dare you twist my words so, and refer to a religion on the same plane as communism? How dare you?"

"I was just asken about adjustments," Gertie said, the words coming more easily, "and what it means."

"You know perfectly well I mean no such thing." Mrs. Whittle bit her freshly lipsticked lips. "The trouble is," she went on, "you don't want to adjust—and Ruben doesn't either."

"That's part way right," Gertie said, moving past her to the stairs. "But he cain't help the way he's made. It's a lot more trouble to roll out steel—and make it like you want it—than it is biscuit dough." (Arnow 1954, pp. 334–335).

In many respects, this passage is about the hegemonic (mainstream) urban institutions and the power urban culture has over rural migrants. It is also about the logical abilities and the sheer intelligence of rural people when they are confronted with the cogs in the urban bureaucratic wheel. When Mrs. Whittle accuses Gertie of not wanting to adjust, and Gertie agrees, Mrs. Whittle understands Gertie's resistance to urban institutions, but for the wrong reasons. That is, she does not understand that before her sits a strong, resilient woman who refuses to give up her rural culture and identity in order to comply with the teacher's demands for her child to "behave" in school. Rather, Mrs. Whittle really believes that "adjustment" is right for Gertie's son and for Gertie herself. Their resistance—and thus their failure to adjust—is, from the teacher's point of view, a weakness. Mrs. Whittle does not understand Ruben's strengths—nor does she understand the strengths of rural Appalachian culture. Gertie, however, does. "Steel" and "biscuit dough" are metaphors for Ruben's resistance to malleability. Gertie sends a verbal bullet right to the teacher who has the power to determine her son's success or failure. She also challenges the teacher's competence to deal with a child who is as strong as her son. In doing so, Gertie challenges the whole system.

The tendency on the part of powerful outsiders to impose judgments on what constitutes adjustment to the city and to advocate that rural people give up their identities and cultures ("our country ways") rather than to allow any kind of negotiation between rural and urban cultures, unfortunately, is all too common. The legal system, the health care system, along with educational systems all work against such negotiating processes; they are time-consuming if nothing else. Some examples are in order. The first involves the health care system; the second pertains to the legal system.

I had the occasion to accompany the adult daughter of an Alzheimer's patient during one of her mother's many stints in an urban teaching hospital. During the course of the hospital stay, both the young resident and the attending physician applied great pressure upon the daughter to place her mother in a nursing home. Although the mother is increasingly incontinent and disoriented and is at times very combative and difficult to handle, her daughter would not consider a nursing home. To place her mother in such a home would be "putting her away," as in a prison. After a great deal of discussion, during which I explained to the resident that intergenerational ties are among the keystones of Appalachian social structure and that placement of elderly relatives in nursing homes is the equivalent of a death sentence, or close to it, home nursing care and an Alzheimer's day care center for three days each week were considered by the health care team. The patient returned home where she can be cared for by her daughter and two neighbors, a mother and her adult daughter. In addition, "grandma," as she is called by her great-granddaughter, receives love and attention from her great-grandbabies. She spends much of her time on her front porch and, especially in good weather, rarely moves from her perch overlooking the neighborhood. She also spends several days each month with her other daughter and her grown children.

The second example involves a mother attempting to defend her young adolescent daughter as the daughter was being charged with complicity in a robbery. The mother, who we will call Tanya, is in her midtwenties and is a speaker of Appalachian English. She and her daughter experienced "real discrimination," according to a neighbor who was also present in the courtroom. When I asked about the nature of the discrimination, the neighbor replied that the people in the courtroom did not know anything about Tanya's neighborhood or about what a good mother Tanya was. In addition, the arresting officer was determined to be harsh largely because of Tanya's daughter's stepfather's misdeeds. The child was placed on probation on condition that any future problems she might have would automatically place her in a correctional home for adolescents. Such institutions are regarded by the community as sentencing children to a lifetime of crime and drug abuse.

In another completely separate case, the great-grandchild of a neighborhood resident was placed in a foster home in an entirely different county. Further, the public defender suggested that the child's mother divorce her husband if she wanted the child back in her home. The only reason given was that the attorney thought the father was a "smart aleck." I have observed and uncovered many such examples of insensitivity to culture and place. All of them point up the blatant hostility of institutions composing the urban power structure.

The idea of reshaping the urban environment and urban institutions to fit the needs of working-class people has not been given nearly enough consideration by policymakers. If education, housing, health care, and social services are to be effective, urban environments must be molded to include community-based services, affordable housing, programs for children and adolescents, and the like.

Bureaucracies may find it more efficient to operate from one central office; however, the cost to communities of having to seek health and social services from outsiders who are strangers is very great. Mental health clinics, social services agencies, and large magnet high schools are only some examples of the kinds of services that have now become so centralized that they cannot service the needs of people in communities in an effective manner. That working-class people resist seeking health and social services from such centralized agencies is not at all surprising. Such resistance only aggravates the problems and increases the costs to society in the long run. Many Appalachians in cities simply do not trust outsiders. To assume that working-class people should, somehow, adjust to the system is to engage in one of the worst forms of ethnocentrism.

DEALING WITH ETHNOCENTRISM

It is critical that every effort be made to neutralize ethnocentrism. Even advocates use terms such as *adjustment, upward mobility,* and *success* in ways that impose ethnocentric judgments on Appalachians in cities. For example, if we look for patterns of success that fit urban, capitalist standards, we may overlook the great strengths of working-class neighborhoods—the intergenerational ties and the informal educational processes that are carried out by older relatives and community people for younger generations as well as the intricate patterns of exchange and gift-giving that ensure both that no one goes hungry or without shelter and that children and the dependent elderly are cared for. When these kin and neighborhood support systems break down, the urban power structure tends to blame the victims or the informal health and child care providers. The urban power structure often fails to comprehend that important community support systems have broken down when there is no one to ask for a ride or to provide temporary housing for people faced with eviction notices. Statistics such as median incomes, school dropout rates, and proportions of renters to owners of homes and apartments do not reflect kin and community-based exchange patterns, informal economies and schooling processes, or the longevity of families in communities. Many Appalachians in cities could have purchased their homes several times over with the amount of rent they have paid; they simply never have had credit lines or the down payments to purchase their homes because they shared their incomes with members of extended family networks and with members of neighborhood networks as well.

It is the responsibility of researchers not merely to uncover these facts of social structure in Appalachian communities but also to help the urban power structure use these facts effectively—that is, for the benefit of people living in working-class communities. This is not an easy task; the urban power structure will use every possible excuse to ignore working-class communities. Also, the mechanisms for working-class representation at city hall, wherever that "hall" may be, are not in place. Token representation on city committees does not mean that community input to such major initiatives as community development programs can be taken for granted. I have seen working-class voices silenced in both blatant and subtle ways. College student interns may fail to record community voices in committee minutes; a committee chair or city official may put down a community person or, at best, treat members of the community in a patronizing fashion. Issues of race and gender also come into play; black Appalachian women have a more difficult time being heard than white Appalachian women; men command more attention than women; and so forth.

The symbols of power are all too evident at city hall—business suits, standard English language, to name two. Without access to these, working-class voices are muted at best. While it may be the case, for example, that members of city council will be advocates for neighborhoods, which neighborhoods receive priority and how information about neighborhood needs and strengths is transmitted to city council members are problematic issues for research and advocacy. Lobbying efforts are necessary, and for working-class people to lobby without advocates/researchers is difficult. This does not mean that advocates and researchers must speak for communities. It does mean that supporting roles are essential; the script for playing these roles has yet to be written, but the roles are first and foremost to be understood as collaborative.

DATA COLLECTION

Researchers and advocates have argued that we need to know more about Appalachian neighborhoods and families (Obermiller 1981). But what exactly do we need to know? Are census tracts and neighborhoods the appropriate units of analysis (Maloney 1987)? Do we know anything about "the symbolic construction of community" (Cohen 1985)? For example, the issue of community boundaries is a highly complicated and symbolic construction. This issue is debated constantly in local community council meetings. We know something about who participates in community councils by the standard socioeconomic indicators, but do we know how community councils work? Do we know how community councils change over time? Do we understand their dynamics and the extraordinary energy required on the part of local leaders to obtain resources for communities? Community council meetings are forums for expressing community conflict, identity, strengths, needs, and weaknesses. Who engenders conflict, who controls it, and which issues are singled out for constant (often filibuster-style) debate are only some of the elements of community council dynamics. Do we understand how much persistence and patience are involved in doing community work in the face of criticism (sometimes bordering on slander) from members of opposing factions within local communities and in the face of constant attempts by wealthier and more powerful outsiders to control local communities? The linkages between local residents and leaders and outsiders are just beginning to be examined for Appalachians in cities (Maloney, Halperin, and Timm, 1993).

The question of units of description and analysis is very complicated. Census takers traditionally have used the household as the unit of analysis. Yet we know that in most urban working-class communities household composition is fluid, and nuclear families are the exceptions rather than the rule. Even where households are occupied by nuclear families, or by single individuals, extended family members are usually very close at hand—in an adjacent apartment, in a house across the street, or, at most, two or three miles away in a neighboring community. Regional ties are important as well, since many Appalachians in cities, even those who are third-, fourth-, or fifth-generation "urbanites," retain ties to relatives in rural areas or to family land outside the city.

COMBATING STEREOTYPES OR CONFIRMING THEM: THE ROLE OF RESEARCHERS IN QUANTITATIVE RESEARCH

It has often been thought to be the task of researchers to counter negative stereotypes that originate with conservative political agendas or with some version of elitist (and urban) ethnocentrism. Negative labels for Appalachians, both rural and urban, have a long history (McCoy and Watkins 1981; Precourt 1983).

It is by no means a given, however, that social scientists or advocates, however well intentioned, are immune from stereotyping or from being perceived by community leaders as damaging community identity or self-image. In the next few pages, I describe a scenario in which the presentation of data from a community survey of what appeared to be "objective" (quantifiable) facts was perceived by community leaders to be damaging to the community and, for a time, resulted in the rejection of two advocacy organizations and their representatives by community leaders. My point here is not to condemn these organizations or their representatives but rather to examine the issues raised by the fact that a qualitative, ethnographic study was welcomed so enthusiastically in the community because it was perceived as "correcting" the misconceptions created by the quantitative study.

In February 1991, shortly before a university-based, ethnographic research project (using in-depth interviews of families and participant observation in the community as a whole and especially at community meetings) was to begin, a report summarizing the results of an earlier survey carried out by two advocacy agencies was presented before the monthly meeting of a community council in a predominantly Appalachian neighborhood in a midwestern city. The community leadership immediately pounced on this report as portraying the community "as a bunch of screaming illiterates." The survey had collected data on levels of school attainment and dropout rates and presented summaries of "the facts" about the community.

There were several ironies: first, as the director of the ethnographic research, I regarded the survey as a necessary and prior step to our qualitative research. That community leaders did not see things this way was initially surprising to me, but I soon realized that the two advocacy agencies sponsoring the survey research had assumed (on the basis of prior track records) their credibility in the neighborhood. Second, the principal investigator of the survey was a key member of our research team—a point we did not emphasize in the community at the beginning of our ethnographic research. We did, however, go to some lengths to improve the image of the entire survey team in the course of the ethnographic research, and we maintained close ties with the members of the survey group.

Our approach to the ethnographic work in the community was very different from that of the survey group. For many months, we walked on eggshells, and very slowly at that. At the time we entered the community, two substantial apartment complexes had been shut down by the city, and their residents had been evicted. Outsiders were particularly suspect in this community since the city was creating a community development plan that, without appropriate community input, could threaten the very existence of the community. The plan had raised fears that people's homes would be taken by the city's right of eminent domain and that additional evictions and displacements would occur.

Having heard many horror stories of anthropologists being thrown out of communities, I felt that the primary task of our research team was to establish our dual roles as researchers and advocates. From the outset, we made it clear to the community leaders in many face-to-face conversations in people's homes, in the local bar, and in the community center that our research was designed to strengthen the voices of community people in the planning process. An additional irony was the fact that our funding was provided by an agency that supported collaborative research between the university and "established" organizations in the city. After assuring the community leaders that all data collected would be confidential, we agreed to share positive community image-building information with the leadership. For example, we found that size of extended families in the neighborhood and the length of residence in the community were no different for renters than for homeowners. Contrary to the conventional wisdom in the city, renters were not transients. Of course, people in the community knew this already; we were merely confirming and legitimizing their knowledge.

As the research proceeded, study team members provided to community leaders advice, moral support, and even, at times, assistance with note taking or typing minutes or letters. Study team members accompanied community council officers and other residents to meetings with developers and city council members and to public hearings with city council or council committees. In the final city council hearings on the plan, the researchers/advocates testified in support of the community.

This account raises many issues for research and for advocacy. What kind of data are most useful to research and to advocacy? Should the ethnographic study have come first? Certainly both the community and the researchers would have benefited from getting to know one another as people rather than as numbers. Since qualitative and quantitative data were collected in the course of the ethnographic research, perhaps the research design should have combined both approaches from the outset. But where do we go from here? Are there research models from other urban ethnographies done in working-class communities? Do other studies of rural urban migrants shed any light on Appalachians in cities? The answer, of course, is yes.

MIGRANTS IN CITIES:
IMPLICATIONS FOR UNITS OF ANALYSIS

In their provocative book *Migrants in Europe*, Hans and Judith-Maria Buechler (1987) have put together a series of case studies of migration to urban areas of Europe that parallel closely the case of Appalachian migrants to cities. This recent work on migration is innovative because it rejects the older, more traditional approach that focused on notions of adaptation, integration, and assimilation in a manner not unlike that of Mrs. Whittle, the teacher in *The Dollmaker*. In place of these rather ethnocentric and simplistic notions, scholars who are studying migrants in cities have begun to examine the shaping of communities and the creativity of migrants in the contexts of regions, nations, and the world system.

One of the most important features of migrants and migration is physical relocation. Too often, however, the assumption is made that people and their families move from place A to place B in a single, unilineal movement that has a beginning, a midpoint, and an end. What is more accurate, and what is certainly true of Appalachians in cities, is that people move in a variety of directions at many different points in time (seasonally, at different points in the life course, periodically, etc.): between rural and urban areas, from one urban community to another, and in some instances, between urban and suburban areas. Let me provide a few illustrations.

Some Appalachians in cities move in and out of rural areas on a regular basis. While the idiom of mobility usually takes the form of a "visit to relatives" or "a trip back home," these folk expressions tell only a small part of the story. People who are relatively well off may own land "up river" and farm it in some capacity. Other people may genuinely need the resources of the rural areas as often as once or twice a month and return regularly to their family land for extended periods. In extreme cases, we may see a bilocal residence pattern in which people return to the rural parts of Appalachia as often as once a month (Halperin 1990). More commonly, however, Appalachian people in cities maintain ties with relatives in rural areas by visiting, exchanging child care on weekends, getting together for holidays, and the like. Children are often among the most mobile. I know of a four-year-old boy who commonly spends at least one night per week with his grandmother; she cares for him during the workweek in an urban area. This child lives in a suburb, but when asked to assert his identity in association with a place, he names the urban, not the suburban, community. Any form of data collection that uses the household as the unit of analysis will miss this kind of residence pattern and the associated cultural identities.

Our units of analysis, then, must be family and community networks, conceived as sets of people connected socially and culturally but not necessarily residentially. It is very important to emphasize several points about the family network here. The first is that the family is not to be understood solely as a biological unit. The family has a biological basis, but if we restricted our definition of family to bonds created by blood or marital ties, we would erase from the analysis many of the most critical relationships for Appalachians in cities. For example, adoption, both formal (legal) and informal, is very common. Relationships between adoptive parents and biological parents often remain close throughout the period of child rearing and into the adopted child's adulthood. Kin networks proliferate as well.

Second, the family is not to be understood as a residential unit, even if we expand the residential unit to the community level. Members of families may reside near one another in the same community, but more commonly, family members spread themselves throughout the region, and they move around in the region and the community with some frequency. The combinations of circumstances faced by the working poor create high rates of geographic mobility both within and between communities. Accidents such as house fires and natural disasters such as tornados and floods combine with the exigencies of substandard housing to cause people to seek alternative residences, both temporary and permanent. Displacement, either by city officials or because of increases in taxes, is another precipitant of mobility.

These are not, as is too often said, signs of instability—social, economic, or cultural. In fact, what remain remarkably in place and stable are the family networks that mobilize to provide food, clothing, and shelter for displaced relatives. Neighborhood networks also play a role here, since the people available to help one another on a daily basis are often coresidents who are not kin. For example, help in taking care of elderly relatives is certainly provided by members of kin networks, but it is also provided by neighbors who live close by. In exchange for elder care, people may receive a variety of forms of payment in cash or in kind. In one instance, a daughter of a frail elderly woman who required constant watching cooks regularly for the caregiver and her mother. In another instance, an elderly woman who is mentally ill has her meals brought to her by members of a neighboring family who worry that she has lost so much weight. These informal support systems are critical to people's survival. They also make up for state support that either is not available or is rejected by many people who would rather care for their kin in their homes and in community contexts.

The fact that people move around in neighborhoods means that a different set of coresidents can be mobilized with each move. Thus, there are, at least potentially, two sources of help for Appalachians in cities: the kin network and the neighborhood network. This last statement assumes that neighborhoods are to some degree intact. Obviously, given too much mobility, caused, for example, by rapid and frequent displacement, neighborhood networks will break down. Family networks are much more resilient in this respect, precisely because they are not residentially based.

THE IMPORTANCE OF THE PAST

Halpern (1987) has noted the importance of the past for Yugoslavian migrants by asserting that the past is in the present. A strong sense of the past is also evident among Appalachian migrants in cities, whether "the past" takes the form of a family history, of recalling past events, or of remembering the community as it was in its prime. Researchers must be extremely careful not to take the current situations of Appalachians in cities as long-standing or permanent; more accurately, Appalachians in cities live under situations of constant change.

It is extremely important to pay attention to several different types of history. Oral histories, for example, are extremely rich sources of insight into social structure, culture, and identity. Many of the oral historians never write their own histories. These histories are complex and varied, and they provide not only windows to the past but also models for the future, especially regarding educational processes (apprenticeships, for example) and processes of community relationships.

The need for thick descriptions that portray the complexity, richness, and creativity of life for Appalachian people in cities is urgent. Little is known about the combinations of livelihood strategies that operate in cities. People on welfare also work at odd jobs, in flea markets, and in the community for landlords and patrons. Indeed, they are paid "under the table." Without such informal economic activities, people and their families would not survive. Another strategy involves the pooling of income and labor among members of extended families.

Family histories that reveal the dynamics of intergenerational relationships in all of their dimensions (education, economic, psychological)—the constant informal mentoring and tutoring, the patience of grandmothers with grandbabies—must be collected. We need as researchers to collect data that avoid the patronizing "we" (urban professionals) who know what is best for "you" or "them" (the poor people). Indeed, urban professionals have a great deal to learn from the working class. If we are to achieve this outcome, community people must be involved with the research from the outset as collaborators. In some respects, this involves legitimizing local knowledge, including common sense. Telling those in power what community people already know and have known for generations is very important. Repackaging the folk wisdom in terms that are understandable to those in positions of power has not been done, to my knowledge. This does not mean that a romantic picture must be painted—merely a picture that is oriented toward people and their lives. Statistics do not lie, but they present only a partial and faceless picture.

DISSEMINATING DATA:
ISSUES OF CONFIDENTIALITY AND ETHICS

One of the major challenges to researchers in urban areas, especially to anthropologists who have access, often, to both personal and political information, is how to maintain the role of community advocate/researcher while at the same time preserving confidentiality. Here the number-crunchers have a much easier time of it. In communities where people know one another over several generations and in communities in which people are easily identifiable, especially to insiders, by their political and community roles, it is difficult to write the ethnography in a personal yet confidential fashion. Again, collaboration between researcher/advocates and community leaders and residents is absolutely essential.

To strike a balance between community voices and anthropological analysis is another delicate task. Ethnographies must be written about Appalachians in cities because—if for no other reason—stereotypes still persist and must be countered. Real people with real families living in real communities must come forward in ethnographic monographs. To date, no such ethnographies exist. There is some urgency for this ethnographic task, for it is unclear how long, given the forces of urbanization and economic development, Appalachian people in cities will be identifiable or recognizable.

References

Abbott, Susan. 1989. "Symptoms of Anxiety and Depression among Eastern Kentucky Adolescents: Insights from Comparative Fieldwork." In *Health in Appalachia: Proceedings of the 1988 Conference on Appalachia*, Lexington: University of Kentucky Appalachian Center.

Adams, Jerome A. Interview by Elizabeth Penn, September 1991.

Alessi, G. J., and J. H. Kaye. 1983. *Behavioral Assessment for School Psychologists*. Washington, DC: National Association of School Psychologists.

Allen, Sudie E., Karth Harben, Cynthia Harris, Barry Johnson, Richard Noegel, and Robert Williams. 1992. *Proceedings of the National Minority Health Conference: Focus on Environmental Contamination*. Atlanta: Agency for Toxic Substances and Disease Registry.

Appalachian Center. 1986. *The Status of Health Care in Appalachian Kentucky*. Lexington: University Press of Kentucky.

Appalachian Regional Commission. 1979. *Report to Congress on Migration*. Washington, DC: Appalachian Regional Commission.

Arnow, Harriet S. 1954. *The Dollmaker*. New York: Macmillan.

Bagby, Jane W., ed. 1990. *Environment in Appalachia: Proceedings of the 1989 Conference on Appalachian*. Lexington: University of Kentucky Appalachian Center.

Bailey, D. B., Jr. 1987. "Collaborative Goal-Setting with Families: Resolving Differences in Values and Priorities for Services." *Topics in Early Childhood Special Education* 7: 59–71.

Bandura, A. 1969. *Principles of Behavior Modification*. New York: Holt, Rinehart and Winston.

——. 1986. *Social Foundations of Thought and Action: A Social Cognitive Theory*. Englewood Cliffs, NJ: Prentice-Hall.

Bangs, Ralph L., and Vijai P. Singh, eds. 1988. *The State of the Region: Economic, Demographic, and Social Trends in Southwestern Pennsylvania.* Pittsburgh: University of Pittsburgh.

Barkman, A. D. 1990. "Formaldehyde Poisoning: An Appalachian Epidemic." In *Environment in Appalachia: Proceedings of the 1989 Conference on Appalachia,* edited by Jane W. Bagby. Lexington: University of Kentucky Appalachian Center.

Barnett, D. W. 1988. "Professional Judgment: A Critical Appriasal." *School Psychology Review* 17: 656–670.

Barnett, D. W., and K. T. Carey. 1992. *Designing Interventions for Preschool Learning and Behavior Problems.* San Francisco: Jossey-Bass.

Barnett, D. W., R. Collins, C. Coulter, M. J. Curtis, K. Ehrhadt, A. Glaser, C. Reyes, S. Stollar, and M. Winston. 1991. "Ethnic Validity: A Review of Concepts, Strategies, and Practices." Work Group on Ethnic Validity, School Psychology Program, University of Cincinnati. Photocopy.

Barnett, D. W., G. M. Macmann, and K. T. Carey. 1992. "Early Intervention and the Assessment of Developmental Skills: Challenges and Directions." *Topics in Early Childhood Special Education* 12 (1): 21–43.

Batteau, Allen. 1983. *Appalachia and America: Autonomy and Regional Dependence.* Lexington: The University Press of Kentucky.

Beaver, P. D. 1979. "Hillbilly Women, Hillbilly Men: Sex Roles in Rural-Agricultural Appalachia." In *Appalachian Women: A Learning /Teaching Guide,* edited by S. B. Lord and C. Patton-Crowder. Newton, MA: Education Development Center.

——. 1988. "Appalachian Cultural Systems, Past and Present." In *Appalachian Mental Health,* edited by S. E. Keefe. Lexington: University Press of Kentucky.

Berea College. n.d. "Newcomers from the Southern Mountains." Berea, KY: Author. Mimeo.

Bijou, S. W., R. F. Peterson, and M. H. Ault. 1968. "A Method to Integrate Descriptive and Experimental Field Studies at the Level of Data and Empirical Concepts." *Journal of Applied Behavior Analysis* 1: 175–91.

Bijou, S. W., R. F. Peterson, F. R. Harris, K. E. Allen, and M. S. Johnston. 1969. "Methodology for Experimental Studies of Young Children in Natural Settings." *The Psychological Record* 19: 177–210.

Bodnar, John, Roger Simon, and Michael P. Weber. 1982. *Lives of Their Own.* Chicago: University of Chicago Press.

Borman, Kathryn M. 1991. *Urban Appalachian Children and Youth at Risk.* Cincinnati: University of Cincinnati.

Borman, Kathryn M., N. S. Lippincott, and C. M. Matey. 1978. "Family and Classroom Control in an Urban Appalachian Neighborhood." *Education and Urban Society* 11: 61–86.

Borman, Kathryn M., E. Mueninghoff, and K. Piazza. 1989. "Urban Appalachian Girls and Young Women: Bowing to No One." In *Class, Race, and Gender in U.S. Schools,* edited by L. Weis. Albany: Sage.

Borman, Kathryn M., S. Piazza, and E. Mueninghoff. 1983. "Lower Price Hill's Children: The Effects of School, Neighborhood, and Family." In *Appalachia and America: Autonomy and Regional Dependence,* edited by Allen Batteau. Lexington: The University Press of Kentucky.

Borman, Kathryn M., and J. H. Spring. 1984. *Schools in Central Cities: Structure and Process.* New York: Longman.

Bornstein, P. H., S. B. Hamilton, and M. T. Bornstein. 1986. "Self-Monitoring Procedures." In *Handbook of Behavioral Assessment,* 2nd ed., edited by A. R. Ciminero, K. S. Calhoun, and H. E. Adams. New York: Wiley.

Bowman, Sr. Elizabeth. 1984. "Religious and Cultural Variety: Gift to Catholic Schools." In *The Non-Catholic in the Catholic School,* edited by F. D. Kelly. Washington, DC: Department of Religious Education, National Catholic Educational Association.

Bramlett, R. K. 1990. "The Development of a Preschool Observation Code: Preliminary Technical Characteristics." Doctoral dissertation, University of Cincinnati.

Bransome, J. 1978. "Appalachian Migrants and the Need for a National Policy." In *Perspectives on Urban Appalachians,* edited by Steven Weiland, Thomas E. Wagner, and Phillip J. Obermiller. Cincinnati: Ohio Urban Appalachian Awareness Project, University of Cincinnati.

Brown, George. 1990. Interview by Phillip J. Obermiller, Hamilton, Ohio.

Brown, James S. 1950. "The Social Organization of an Isolated Kentucky Mountain Neighborhood." Doctoral dissertation, Harvard University.

Brown, James S., and George A. Hillery. 1962. "The Great Migration 1940–1960." In *The Southern Appalachian Region: A Survey,* edited by Thomas R. Ford. Lexington: University of Kentucky Press.

——. 1972. "A Look at the 1970 Census." In *Appalachia in the Sixties: A Decade of Reawakening,* edited by David Walls and John Stephenson. Lexington: University of Kentucky Press.

Brown, K., and Phillip J. Obermiller. 1990. "The Health Status of Children Living in Urban Appalachian Neighborhoods." Paper presented at meeting of the International Society for Environmental Epidemiology, Berkeley.

Bryant, B., and P. Mohai, eds. 1992. *Race and the Incidence of Environmental Hazards: A Time for Discourse.* Boulder: Westview.

Buechler, Hans, and Judith-Maria Buechler. 1987. *Migrants in Europe: The Role of Family, Labor, and Politics.* New York: Greenwood.

Bullard, Robert F. 1983. "Solid Waste Sites and the Houston Black Community." *Sociological Inquiry* 53: 273–88.

——. 1990a. *Dumping in Dixie: Race, Class and Environmental Quality.* Boulder: Westview.

——. 1990b. "Environmentalism, Economic Blackmail, and Civil Rights: Competing Agendas in the Black Community." In *Communities in Economic Crisis: Appalachia and the South,* edited by John Gaventa, Barbara Smith, and Alex Willingham. Philadelphia: Temple University Press.

——, ed. 1992. *Confronting Environmental Racism: Voices from the Grassroots.* Boston: South End Press.

Bullard, Robert F., and Beverly H. Wright. 1985. "The Politics of Pollution: Implications for the Black Community." *Phylon* 47: 71–8.

——. 1987a. "Blacks and the Environment." *Humboldt Journal of Social Relations* 14: 65–84.

——. 1987b. "Environmentalism and the Politics of Equity: Trends in the Black Community." *Mid-American Review of Sociology* 12: 21–38.

Buttel, Frederick R., and William L. Flinn. 1978. "Social Class and Mass Environmental Beliefs: A Reconsideration." *Environment and Behavior* 10: 433–50.

CACI Marketing Systems. 1985. "Geography Source Diskette." Fairfax, VA: author.

Campbell, J. C. 1921. *The Southern Highlander and His Homeland.* Lexington: University Press of Kentucky.

Campinha-Bacote, J. 1991. Interview by Kathryn M. Borman, Cincinnati, Ohio.

Catchen, James. 1989. Interview by Phillip J. Obermiller, Covington, Kentucky.

Center for Appalachian Studies and Services. 1989. "Sense of Place in Appalachia." *Now and Then Special Issue* 6 (1).

Chestang, L. 1982. "Review of *The Ethnic Dilemma in Social Services* by Shirley Jenkins." *Social Work* 27 (1): 117.

Children's Defense Fund. 1990. *The Nation's Investment in Children.* Washington, DC: author.

Cleaver, Eldridge. 1969. *Eldridge Cleaver: Post Prison Writings and Speeches*. New York: Knopf.

Cohen, Anthony P. 1985. *The Symbolic Construction of Community*. London: Tavistock.

Coles, Robert. 1971. *The South Goes North*. Boston: Little, Brown.

Commission for Racial Justice. 1987. *Toxic Waste and Race in the United States*. Cleveland: United Church of Christ.

Community Chest and Council of the Cincinnati Area. 1983. "Essay on Minority Populations." In *Regional Overview Report II: Profiles of Change in the Greater Cincinnati Region*. Cincinnati: Community Chest.

Council of the Southern Mountains. 1965. *Are You Thinking of Moving to the City?* Berea, KY: Council of the Southern Mountains.

Courts, P. 1991. *Literacy and Empowerment*. New York: Bergin and Garvey.

Couto, R. 1978. "Prophets in Health Care." *Southern Exposure* 6: 72–79.

——. 1983. "Appalachian Innovations in Health Care." In *Appalachia and American: Autonomy and Regional Dependence,* edited by Allen Batteau. Lexington: University Press of Kentucky.

Cutter, Susan C. 1981. "Community Concern for Pollution: Social and Environmental Influences." *Environment and Behavior* 13: 105–24.

Dahl, K., V., Purcell-Gates, and E. McIntyre. 1989. *An Investigation of the Way Low SES Learners Make Sense of Instruction in Reading and Writing in the Early Grades*. Final Report to the U.S. Department of Education, Office of Educational Research and Information: Grant No. G008720229. Washington, DC: Department of Education.

Damberg, C. L. 1986. "Strategies for Promoting the Health of Minorities: The School-Age Population." *Health Values* 10: 29–33.

Davidson, L. and L. K. Gordon. 1979. *The Sociology of Gender*. Chicago: Rand McNally.

Delgado, Gary. 1986. *Toxics and Minority Communities*. Oakland: Alternative Policy Institute of the Center for Third World Organizing.

De Soto, Hernando. 1989. *The Other Path*. New York: Harper & Row.

DeStefano, Johanna S. 1989. "Literacy Learning and Cultural Conflict: The Case of Tom, Dick and Harry." In *Festschrift in Honor of Georgi Kostic*, edited by S. Viadisavjevic. Belgrade: The Institute of Experimental Phonetics.

——. 1990. "Assessing Students' Communicative Competence Using a Linguistic Analysis Procedure." In *Linguistics and Education* 2: 127–145.

——. 1991. "Ethnolinguistic Minority Groups and Literacy: Tom, Dick and Harry at Home and in School." In *Language in School and Society: Policy and Pedagogy,* edited by M. McGroarty and C. Faltis. New York: Mouton de Gruyter.

DeStefano, Johanna S., H. B. Pepinsky, and T. S. Sanders. 1982. "Discourse Rules for Literacy Learning in a Classroom." In *Communicating in the Classroom,* edited by L. Cherry-Wilkinson. New York: Academic Press.

Dillard, J. M. 1983. "Southern Appalachian Anglo Americans." In *Multi-cultural Counseling.* Chicago: Nelson-Hall.

Drake, Charles. 1960. "Migration Myths." Berea, KY: Council of the Southern Mountains. Mimeo.

Dunst, C. J., and C. M. Trivette. 1987. "Enabling and Empowering Families: Conceptual and Intervention Issues." *School Psychology Review* 16: 443–56.

Dunst, C. J., C. M. Trivette, and A. H. Cross. 1988. "Social Support Networks of Families with Handicapped Children. In *Appalachian Mental Health* edited by S. E. Keefe. Lexington, KY: University Press of Kentucky.

Edelstein, Michael R. 1987. *Contaminated Communities: The Social and Psychological Impacts of Residential Toxic Exposure.* Boulder: Westview.

Education for All Handicapped Children Act. 1975. Public Law 94–142.

Egan, Rosemary. 1977. *Interpreting Testing Data.* St. Louis: Milliken.

Elkind, D. 1979. *The Child and Society.* New York: Oxford University Press.

"EPA Debates Minority Protection: Group To Check for Racism in Rule-making." 1992. *Cincinnati Enquirer,* February 25, A4.

"EPA Has a New Emphasis: Agencies Looking Out for Interests of Minorities, Poor." 1992. *Cincinnati Enquirer,* January 21, A8.

Ergood, Bruce, and Bruce Kuhre, eds. 1991. *Appalachia: Social Context Past and Present,* 3rd ed. Dubuque: Kendall Hunt.

Erickson, D. 1981. "The Superior Social Climate of Private Schools." *Momentum* 12 (4): 5–8.

Fawcett, S. B., R. M. Mathews, and R. K. Fletcher. 1980. "Some Promising Dimensions for Behavioral Community Technology." *Journal of Applied Behavior Analysis* 13: 505–18.

Fisher, Stephen. 1986. "The Nicaraguan Revolution and the U.S. Response: Lessons for Appalachia." *Appalachian Journal* 14: 22–37.

Flory, Dan. 1990. Interview by Phillip J. Obermiller, Cincinnati, Ohio.

Ford, Thomas R., ed. 1962. *The Southern Appalachian Region: A Survey.* Lexington: University of Kentucky Press.

Fowler, Gary L. 1981. "The Residential Distribution of Urban Appalachians." In *The Invisible Minority: Urban Appalachians,* edited by William W. Philliber and Clyde B. McCoy. Lexington: University Press of Kentucky.

Fowler, Gary L., and Christopher S. Davies. 1972. "The Urban Settlement Patterns of Disadvantaged Migrants." *Journal of Geography* 17: 275–84.

Friedl, J. 1978. *Health Care Services and the Appalachian Migrant.* Columbus: The Ohio State University Press.

——. 1983. "Health Care: The City Versus the Migrant." In *Appalachia and America: Autonomy and Regional Dependence* edited by Allen Batteau. Lexington: University Press of Kentucky.

Fruend, D. A. 1984. "Equality of Opportunity and the Demand for Medical Care by Race." *Quarterly Review of Economics and Business* 24: 42–55.

Galli, N., J. S. Greenberg, and F. Tobin. 1987. "Health Education and Sensitivity to Cultural, Religious, and Ethnic Beliefs." *Journal of School Health* 57: 177–80.

Gans, Herbert. 1962. *The Urban Villagers.* Glencoe: The Free Press.

——. 1992. "Fighting the Biases Embedded in Social Concepts of the Poor." *Chronicle of Higher Education,* January, A56.

Gerber, M. M., and M. I. Semmel. 1984. "Teacher as Imperfect Test: Reconceptualizing the Referral Process." *Exceptional Children* 54: 309–14.

Gibbard, Harold A. 1962. "Extractive Industries and Forestry." In *The Southern Appalachian Region: A Survey,* edited by T. R. Ford. Lexington: University of Kentucky Press.

Giffin, Roscoe. 1954. "Report of a Workshop on the Southern Mountaineer in Cincinnati." Cincinnati: Mayor's Friendly Relations Committee and the Social Service Association of Cincinnati. Mimeo.

——. 1978. "From Cinder Hollow to Cincinnati." In *Perspectives on Urban Appalachians,* edited by Steven Weiland and Phillip J. Obermiller. Cincinnati: Ohio Urban Appalachian Awareness Project, University of Cincinnati.

Goldin, B. 1990. *Everyday People.* Austin: Steck-Vaughn.

Green, J. W. 1982. *Cultural Awareness in the Human Services.* Englewood Cliffs, NJ: Prentice-Hall.

Greene, L. W., et al. 1980. *Health Education Planning: A Diagnostic Approach.* Palo Alto: Mayfield.

Gutkin, T. B., and M. J. Curtis. 1982. "School-based Consultation: Theory and Techniques." In *The Handbook of School Psychology,* edited by C.R. Reynolds and T.B. Gutkin. New York: Wiley.

Hager, Lora Lea. 1989. "A Death in the Family." *Goldenseal* 15: 7.

Halperin, Rhoda. 1990. *The Livelihood of Kin*. Austin: University of Texas Press.

Halpern, Joel. 1987. "Yugoslav Migration Process and Employment in Western Europe: A Historical Perspective." In *Migrants in Europe: The Role of Family, Labor, and Politics*, edited by Hans Buechler and Judith-Maria Buechler. New York: Greenwood.

Hamilton, C. H. 1962. "Health and Health Services." In *The Southern Appalachian Region: A Survey,* edited by T. R. Ford. Lexington: University of Kentucky Press.

Hamilton, Lawrence. 1985. "Concern about Toxic Waste: Three Demographic Predictors." *Sociological Perspective* 28: 463–86.

Hart, B. 1985. "Naturalistic Language Training Techniques." In *Teaching Functional Language,* edited S. F. Warren and A. Rogers-Warren. Austin: Pro Ed.

Hayes, Arthur S. 1992. "Environmental Poverty Specialty Helps Poor Fight Pollution." *Wall Street Journal*, October 9, B5.

Heath, S. B. 1983. *Ways with Words: Language, Life and Work in Communities and Classrooms*. Cambridge: Cambridge University Press.

Horowitz, D. L. 1975. "Ethnic Identity." In *Ethnicity: Theory and Experience*, edited by Glazer and D. Moynihan. Cambridge: Harvard University Press.

Howe, Howard, II. 1991. "Seven Large Questions for America 2000's Authors." In *Voices from the Field*. Washington, DC: Wm. T. Grant Foundation Commission on Work, Family and Citizenship.

Howell, Joseph. 1973. *Hard Living on Clay Street*. Garden City, NY: Anchor.

——. 1978. "Appalachian Values." In *Perspectives on Urban Appalachia,* edited by Steven Weiland and Phillip J. Obermiller. Cincinnati: Ohio Urban Appalachian Awareness Project, University of Cincinnati.

Jones, L. 1975. "Appalachian Values." In *Voices from the Hills*, edited by R. Higgs and A. Manning. New York: Frederick Unger.

Kahn, Kathy. 1973. *Hillbilly Women*. New York: Doubleday.

Kanamine, Linda. 1992. "Born Victims: Babies' Deaths a Mystery." *USA Today*, February 18, 3A.

Kanfer, F. H., and L. G. Grimm. 1977. "Behavior Analysis: Selecting Target Behaviors in the Interview. *Behavior Modification* 1: 7–28.

Keefe, S. E., ed. 1988. *Appalachian Mental Health*. Lexington: University Press of Kentucky.

——. 1988a. "Factors Affecting the Use of Mental Health Services: A Review." In *Appalachian Mental Health*.

——. 1988b. "Appalachian Family Ties." In *Appalachian Mental Health.*

——. 1988c. "Introduction." In *Appalachian Mental Health.*

Kemme, Steve. 1990. "Graying Appalachia Ready to Rest." *Cincinnati Enquirer*, March 4, B6.

Kentucky Department of Education. 1991. *Minorities in Teacher Education Programs.* Frankfort, KY: author.

Kessler, William. 1991. *The Appalachian Environment: Protecting Our Air, Land, and Water.* Lexington and Berea, KY: Appalachian Civic Leadership Project.

Kleinman, A., L. Eisenberg, and B. Good. 1978. "Culture, Illness and Care: Clinical Lessons from Anthropologic and Cross Cultural Research. *Annals of Internal Medicine* 88: 251–58.

Kolodner, Mrs. Fred. 1961. "The Unaccepted Baltimoreans: A Report on the White Southern Rural Migrants." Baltimore: Baltimore Section of the National Council of Jewish Women. Mimeo.

Labonte, R. 1986. "Social Inequality and Healthy Public Policy." *Health Promotion* 1: 341–51.

Levin, L. 1987. "Every Silver Lining Has a Cloud: The Limits of Health Promotion." *Social Policy* (Summer): 57–60.

Lewis, Helen, Linda Johnson, and Don Askins. 1978. *Colonialism in Modern America: The Appalachian Case.* Boone, NC: Appalachian Consortium Press.

Lewis, O. 1961. *The Children of Sanchez.* New York: Random House.

Lincoln, Y. S., and E. G. Guba. 1985. *Naturalistic Inquiry.* Beverly Hills: Sage.

"Living with Pollution: Poverty's Silent Partner." 1991. *Greenpeace Magazine* October–December: 8–13.

Loof, David H. 1971. *Appalachia's Children: The Challenge of Mental Health.* Lexington: University Press of Kentucky.

Lord, S. B., and C. Patton-Crowder. 1979. *Appalachian Women: A Learning/Teaching Guide.* Newton, MA: Educational Development Center.

Lower Price Hill Task Force. 1990. "Report on Health, Education, and Pollution in Lower Price Hill." Cincinnati: Urban Appalachian Council. Mimeo.

Mabry, C. Charlton, 1989. "Children: The Vulnerable Population of Appalachia." In *Health in Appalachia: Proceedings of the 1988 Conference on Appalachia.* Lexington: University of Kentucky Appalachian Center.

McCarthy, John D., and Mayer N. Zald. 1973. *The Trend of Social Movements in America: Professionalization and Resource Mobilization.* Morristown, NJ: General Learning Press.

McCaull, Julian. 1976. "Discriminatory Air Pollution: If the Poor Don't Breathe." *Environment* 19: 26–32.

McCormick, John. 1989. *Reclaiming Paradise: The Global Environmental Movement.* Bloomington: Indiana University Press.

McCoy, Clyde B., and James S. Brown. 1981. "Appalachian Migration to Midwestern Cities." In *The Invisible Minority: Urban Appalachians,* edited by William W. Philliber and Clyde B. McCoy. Lexington: The University Press of Kentucky.

McCoy, Clyde B., and H. McCoy. 1987. "Appalachian Youth in Cultural Transition." In *Too Few Tomorrows: Urban Appalachians in the 1980s,* edited by Phillip J. Obermiller and William W. Philliber. Boone, NC: Appalachian Consortium Press.

McCoy, Clyde B., and Virginia McCoy Watkins. 1980. "Drug Use among Urban Ethnic Youth: Appalachian and Other Comparisons." *Youth and Society:* 83–106.

———. 1981. "Stereotypes of Appalachian Migrants." In *The Invisible Minority: Urban Appalachians,* edited by William W. Philliber and Clyde B. McCoy. Lexington: University Press of Kentucky.

McDiarmid, G. Williamson. 1990. "What To Do about Differences? A Study of Multicultural Education for Teacher Trainees in the Los Angeles Unified School District." East Lansing: National Center for Research on Teacher Education, Michigan State University.

McKee, Dan, and Phillip J. Obermiller. 1978. "From Mountain to Metropolis: Urban Appalachians in Ohio." In *Perspectives on Urban Appalachians,* edited by Steven Weiland, Thomas E. Wagner, and Phillip J. Obermiller. Cincinnati: Ohio Urban Appalachian Awareness Project, University of Cincinnati.

McKenry, P. C., H. M. Reed, and J. L. Knipers. 1979. "Some Perceptions of Family Functioning among Rural Families in East Tennessee." In *Appalachian Women,* edited by S. B. Lord and C. Patton-Crowder. Newton, MA: Educational Development Center.

Maloney, Michael E. 1974a. *The Social Areas of Cincinnati: Towards an Analysis of Social Needs.* Cincinnati: Cincinnati Human Relations Commission.

———. 1974b. *The Prospects for Urban Appalachians,* edited by William W. Philliber and Clyde B. McCoy. Lexington: University Press of Kentucky.

———. 1981. "The Prospects for Urban Appalachians." In *The Invisible Minority: Urban Appalachians,* edited by William W. Philliber and Clyde B. McCoy. Lexington: University Press of Kentucky.

———. 1985. *The Social Areas of Cincinnati: An Analysis of Social Needs,* 2nd ed. Cincinnati: Cincinnati Human Relations Commission.

——. 1987. "A Decade in Review: The Development of the Ethnic Model in Urban Appalachian Studies." In *Too Few Tomorrows: Urban Appalachians in the 1980s,* edited by Phillip J. Obermiller and William W. Philliber. Boone, NC: Appalachian Consortium Press.

——, et al. 1989. *The Moraine School District: A Report.* Cincinnati: Applied Information Resources.

Maloney, Michael E., and Kathryn M. Borman. 1987. "Effects of School and Schooling upon Appalachian Children in Cincinnati." In *Too Few Tomorrows: Urban Appalachians in the 1980s,* edited by Phillip J. Obermiller and William W. Philliber. Boone, NC: Appalachian Consortium Press.

Maloney, Michael G., Rhoda H. Halperin, and Pat Z. Timm. 1993. "A Collaborative Model for Understanding Culture and Practice: An Urban Appalachian Example." Photocopy.

Marger, Martin, and Phillip J. Obermiller. 1983. "Urban Appalachians and Canadian Maritime Migrants: A Comparative Study of Emergent Ethnicity." *International Journal of Comparative Sociology* 24: 229–43.

Meade, Edward J., Jr. 1991. "Ignoring the Lessons of Previous School Reform." In *Voices from the Field: 30 Expert Opinions on America 2000.* Washington, DC: Wm. T. Grant Foundation Commission on Work, Family, and Citizenship and Institute for Educational Leadership.

Meeker, J. W., W. K. Woods, and W. Lucas. 1973. "Red, White, and Black in the National Parks." *North American Review* 258 (3): 3.

Meunninghoff, E., and Kathryn M. Borman. 1982. "Work Roles and Social Roles in Three Elementary School Settings." Paper presented at the American Educational Research Association Annual Meeting, New York, April 1982.

Meyer, Judith W., and Ellen K. Cromley. 1989. "Caregiving Environments and Elderly Residential Mobility." *Professional Geographer* 41: 440–50.

Miles, E. B. 1905. *The Spirit of the Mountains.* Knoxville: University of Tennessee Press.

Miller, Jim Wayne. 1977, 1978, 1979. "Appalachian Values/American Values: The Role of Regional Colleges and Universities." *Appalachian Heritage* 5 (4): 24–32; 6 (1): 30–37; 6 (2): 11–19; 6 (3): 23–34; 6 (4): 47–54; and 7 (1): 49–57.

Miller, M. 1981. *It's a Living.* New York: Basic Books.

Miller, T. 1978. "Urban Appalachian Ethnic Identity: The Current Situation." In *Perspectives on Urban Appalachians,* edited by Steven Weiland, Thomas E. Wagner, and Phillip J. Obermiller. Cincinnati:

Ohio Urban Appalachian Awareness Project, University of Cincinnati.

Minkler, M., and R. Passick. 1986. "Health Promotion and the Elderly: A Critical Perspective on the Past and the Future." In *Wellness and Health Promotion for the Elderly,* edited by K. Dychtwald and J. MacLean. Rockwell, MD: Aspen Publications.

"Minorities Exposed More to Pollution, EPA Reports; Procedures Under Review." 1992. *El Paso Times,* February 25, p.1A.

Mitford, Jessica. 1963. *The American Way of Death.* New York: Simon and Schuster.

Mitchell, Robert C. 1979. "Silent Spring/Solid Majorities." *Public Opinion* 2: 16–20.

——, ed. 1980. "Public Opinion on Environmental Issues." In *The Eleventh Annual Report of the Council on Environmental Quality.* Washington, DC: U.S. Government Printing Office.

——. 1984. "Public Opinion and Environmental Politics in the 1970s and 1980s." In *Environmental Policy in the 1980s: Reagan's New Agenda*, edited by Norman J. Vig and Michael E. Kraft. Washington, DC: Congressional Quarterly Press.

Mohai, Paul. 1985. "Public Concern and Elite Involvement in Environmental-Conservation Issues." *Social Science Quarterly* 66: 820–38.

Montell, William L. 1975. *Ghosts along the Cumberland: Deathlore in the Kentucky Foothills.* Knoxville: University of Tennessee Press.

Morrison, Denton E. 1986. "How and Why Environmental Consciousness Has Trickled Down." In *Distributional Conflict in Environmental-Resource Policy*, edited by Allan Schnaiberg, Nicholas Watts, and Klaus Zimmerman. New York: St. Martin's.

Morrison, Denton E., and Riley E. Dunlap. 1986. "Environmentalism and Elitism: A Conceptual and Empirical Analysis." *Environmental Management* 10: 581–89.

Nathan, Joe, and Jim Kielsmeier. 1991. "The Sleeping Giant of School Reform." *Phi Delta Kappan* (June): 739–42.

National Directory of Morticians. 1989. Chagrin Falls, OH.

Neely, Sharlotte, 1979. "The Urban Appalachian Ethnic Movement." Paper presented at annual meeting of the American Anthropological Association, Cincinnati.

——. 1987. "The Ethnic Entrepreneur in the Urban Appalachian Community." In *Too Few Tomorrows: Urban Appalachians in the 1980s,* edited by Phillip J. Obermiller and William W. Philliber. Boone, NC: Appalachian Consortium Press.

Nelson, Ken. 1988. "Minnesota's Youth Development Initiative: Building on Strengths." *Community Education Journal* (October): 5.

Nesbit, R. 1972. *Social Change*. New York: Harper & Row.

Nugent, K. E., et al. 1988. "A Model for Providing Health Maintenance and Promotion to Children from Low-Income Ethnically Diverse Backgrounds." *Journal of Pediatric Care* 4: 175–80.

Obermiller, Phillip J. 1977. "Appalachians as an Urban Ethnic Group: Romance, Renaissance, or Revolution?" *Appalachian Journal* 5: 145–152.

——. 1978. "On the Question of Appalachian Ethnicity." In *Perspectives on Urban Appalachians*, edited by Steven Weiland and Phillip J. Obermiller. Cincinnati: Ohio Urban Appalachian Awareness Project, University of Cincinnati.

——. 1981. "The Question of Appalachian Ethnicity." In *The Invisible Minority: Urban Appalachians,* edited by William W. Philliber, and Clyde B. McCoy. Lexington, KY: University of Kentucky Press.

——. 1987. "Labeling Urban Appalachians" In *Too Few Tomorrows: Urban Appalachians in the 1980s*, edited by Phillip J. Obermiller and William W. Philliber. Boone, NC: Appalachian Consortium Press.

——. 1991. "Ain't Goin' Back: The Aging of Appalachian Migrants in Urban Neighborhoods." In *Change in the Mountains: Elderly Migration and Population Dynamics in Appalachia*, Occasional Paper Number 2, edited by Graham D. Rowles and John F. Watkins. Lexington, KY: Sanders-Brown Center on Aging, University of Kentucky.

Obermiller, Phillip J., and Michael E. Maloney. 1990a. "Looking for Appalachians in Pittsburgh: Seeking Deliverance, Finding the Deerhunter." *Pittsburgh History* 73: 160–170.

——. 1990b. "The Current Status and Future Prospects of Urban Appalachians." *The Urban Appalachian Advocate* 2 (December).

——. 1991. "Living City, Feeling Country." In *Appalachia: Social Context Past and Present*, 3rd ed., edited by Bruce Ergood and Bruce Kuhre. Dubuque: Kendall Hunt.

Obermiller, Phillip J., and Robert W. Oldendick. 1987. "Moving On: Recent Patterns of Appalachian Migration." In *Too Few Tomorrows: Urban Appalachians in the 1980s*, edited by Phillip J. Obermiller and William W. Philliber. Boone, NC: Appalachian Consortium.

——. 1989. "Urban Appalachian Health Concerns." In *Health in Appalachia: Proceedings of the 1988 University of Kentucky Conference on Appalachia*. Lexington: Appalachian Center.

Obermiller, Phillip J., and William W. Philliber, eds. 1987. *Too Few Tomorrows: Urban Appalachians in the 1980s.* Boone, NC: Appalachian Consortium Press.

Ogbu, J. U. 1988. "Opportunity Structures, Cultural Boundaries and Literacy." In *Language Literacy and Culture: Issues of Society and Schooling,* edited by J. Langer. Norwood, NJ: Ablex.

"Old Time Burials." 1973. In *Foxfire 2,* edited by Eliot Wigginton. Garden City, NY: Anchor.

Opie, John. 1977. "A Sense of Place: The World We Have Lost." In *An Appalachian Symposium,* edited by J.W. Williamson. Boone, NC: Appalachian State University Press.

Osborne, G. L., et al. 1990. "Birth Defects and Pollution: A Study of Spina Bifida in Appalachian Tennessee." In *Environment in Appalachia: Proceedings of the 1989 Conference on Appalachia,* edited by Jane W. Bagby. Lexington: University of Kentucky Appalachian Center.

Pearsall, M. 1960. "Healthways in a Mountain County." *Mountain Life and Work* 36: 7–13.

Peterson, D. R. 1968. *The Clinical Study of Social Behavior.* New York: Appleton Century Crofts.

Philliber, William W. 1981a. "Accounting for the Occupational Placement of Appalachian Migrants." In *The Invisible Minority: Urban Appalachians,* edited by William W. Philliber and Clyde B. McCoy. Lexington: University Press of Kentucky.

——. 1981b. *Appalachian Migrants in Urban America: Cultural Conflict or Ethnic Group Formation?* New York: Praeger.

——. 1987. "The Changing Composition of Appalachian Migrants." In *Too Few Tomorrows: Urban Appalachians in the 1980s* edited by Phillip J. Obermiller and William W. Philliber. Boone, NC: Appalachian Consortium Press.

Philliber, William W., and Clyde B. McCoy. 1981. *The Invisible Minority: Urban Appalachians.* Lexington: University Press of Kentucky.

Philliber, William W., and Phillip J. Obermiller. 1982. "Black Appalachian Migrants: The Issue of Dual Minority Status." In *Critical Essays in Appalachian Life and Culture,* edited by R. Simon. Boone, NC: Appalachian Consortium Press.

Phipps, William E. 1989. *Cremation Concerns.* Springfield, IL: Thomas.

Photiadis, J. D. 1981. "Occupational Adjustments of Appalachians in Cleveland." In *The Invisible Minority: Urban Appalachians,* edited by William W. Philliber and Clyde B. McCoy. Lexington: University Press of Kentucky.

Plaut, T. 1988. "Cross-Cultural Conflict between Providers and Clients and Staff Members." In *Appalachian Mental Health*, edited by S. E. Keefe. Lexington, KY: University Press of Kentucky.

Polansky, N. A., R. D. Borgman, and C. DeSaix. 1972. *Roots of Futility*. San Francisco: Jossey-Bass.

Porter, E. R. 1961. Modern Medicine and the Migrated Mountaineer. *Cincinnati Journal of Medicine* 42: 433–44.

———. 1963a. "When Cultures Meet—Mountain and Urban." *Nursing Outlook* 11: 418–20.

———. 1963b. "From Mountain Folk to City Dwellers." *Nursing Outlook* 11: 514–15.

Powles, W. E. 1964. "The Southern Appalachian Migrant: Country Boy Turned Blue-Collarite." In *Blue Collar World: Studies of the American Worker*, edited by A. Shostak and W. Gomberg. Englewood Cliffs, NJ: Prentice-Hall.

———. 1978. "The Southern Appalachian Migrant: Country Boy Turned Blue-Collarite." In *Perspectives on Urban Appalachians,* edited by Steven Weiland and Phillip J. Obermiller. Cincinnati: Ohio Urban Appalachian Awareness Project, University of Cincinnati.

Precourt, W. 1983. "The Image of Appalachian Poverty." In *Appalachian and American: Autonomy and Regional Dependence*, edited by Allen Batteau. Lexington: University Press of Kentucky.

Proctor, Roy E. and T. Kelley White. 1962. "Agriculture: A Reassessment." In *The Southern Appalachian Region: A Survey*, edited by T. R. Ford. Lexington, KY: University of Kentucky Press.

Qualls, Roxanne. 1991. *Our Industrial Neighbors: The Good, The Bad, and The Ugly*. Cincinnati: Ohio Citizen Action. Mimeo.

Reese, L., C. Goldenbert, J. Loucky, and R. Gallimore. 1989. "Ecocultural Context, Cultural Activity, and Emerging Literacy: Sources of Variation in Home Literacy Experiences of Spanish-Speaking Children." Paper presented at meeting of the American Anthropological Association, Washington, DC.

Riggs, William. 1990. Interview by Phillip J. Obermiller, Middletown, Ohio.

Roncker, Robert. 1959. "The Southern Appalachian Migrant." Cincinnati: Cincinnati Division of Police. Mimeo.

Rowles, Graham D. 1983. "Between Worlds: A Relocation Dilemma for the Appalachian Elderly." *International Journal of Aging and Human Development* 17: 301–14.

———. 1987. "A Place to Call Home." In *Handbook of Clinical Gerontology*, edited by Laura Carstensen and Barry Edelstein. New York: Pergamon.

Rowles, Graham D. and Malcom L. Comeaux. 1986. "Returning Home: The Interstate Transportation of Human Remains." *Omega* 17: 103–13.

——. 1987. "A Final Journey: Post-death Removal of Human Remains." *Journal of Economic and Social Geography* 78: 114–24.

Rutter, M. Maughan, P. Mortimore, and J. Ouston. 1979. *Fifteen Thousand Hours: Secondary Schools and Their Effects on Children.* Cambridge: Harvard University Press.

Savage, J. E., and A. V. Adair. 1980. "Testing Minorities: Developing More Culturally Relevant Assessment Systems." In *Black Psychology*, 2nd ed., edited by R. L. Jones. New York: Harper & Row.

Schon, D. A. 1983. *The Reflective Practitioner: How Professionals Think in Action.* New York: Basic Books.

Schwarzweller, H. 1981. "Occupational Patterns of Appalachian Migrants." In T*he Invisible Minority: Urban Appalachians*, edited by William W. Philliber and Clyde B. McCoy. Lexington: University Press of Kentucky.

Schwarzweller, H., J. S. Brown, and J. Mangalam. 1971. *Mountain Families in Transition.* University Park: Pennsylvania State University Press.

Shneidman, Edwin S. 1976. *Death: Current Perspectives.* Palo Alto: Mayfield.

Sloan, Lester. 1992. "Dumping: A New Form of Genocide?" *Emerge* 3: 19–20.

Smith, Barbara. 1988. "The Family Cemetery: At the Heart of the American Attitude toward Death." In *Sense of Place in Appalachia*, edited by S. Mont Whitson. Morehead, KY: Office of Development Services, Morehead State University.

Snow, C., and A. Ninio. 1986. "The Contacts of Literacy: What Children Learn from Learning to Read Books." In *Emerging Literacy: Writing and Reading*, edited by W. H. Teale and E. Sulzby. Norwood, NJ: Ablex.

Spradley, J. P., and D. W. McCurdy. 1984. *Conformity and Conflict.* Boston: Little, Brown.

Stafford, Chris. 1979. *Say That You Love Me...A Teacher's Guide to Appalachian Awareness.* Cincinnati: Cincinnati Association for the Education of Young Children.

Starnes, B. 1990. "Appalachian Students, Parents and Culture as Viewed by Their Teachers." *Urban Appalachian Advocate* 1: 1–4.

Stegelin, D. 1992. *Early Childhood Education: Policy Issues for the 1990s.* Norwood, NJ: Ablex.

Sticht, T. G. 1973. "Research Toward the Design, Development, and Evaluation of a Job-Functional Literacy Program for the U.S. Army." *Literacy Discussion* 4 (3): 339–369.

Syme, S. L., and L. Berkman. 1976. "Social Class: Susceptibility and Sickness." *American Journal of Epidemiology* 104: 1–8.

Tabachnick, B. G., and L. S. Fidell. 1983. *Using Multivariate Statistics.* New York: Harper & Row.

Taylor, Dorceta E. 1989. "Blacks and the Environment: Toward an Explanation of the Concern and Action Gap between Blacks and Whites." *Environment and Behavior* 21: 175–205.

Taylor, Ronald A. 1984. "Do Environmentalists Care about Poor People?" *U.S. News and World Report*, April 2, 51–2.

Terris, M. 1986. "What is Health Promotion?" *Journal of Public Policy* 7: 147–51.

Traina, F. J. 1980. "The Assimilation of Appalachian Migrants in Northern Kentucky." Cincinnati: Urban Appalachian Council.

Trevino, D. 1978. "Appalachian Women." In *Teaching Mountain Children,* edited by David N. Mielke. Boone, NC: Appalachian Consortium Press.

Tripp-Reimer, T., and M. C. Friedl. 1977. "Appalachians: A Neglected Minority." *Nursing Clinics of North America* 12: 41–54.

Tyson, Rae. 1991. "Target of Toxins? Poor Communities Charge 'Environmental Racism.'" *USA Today*, October 24, 1A, 2A.

Uhlenberg, Peter. 1975. "Noneconomic Determinants of Nonmigration: Sociological Considerations of Migration Theory." *Rural Sociology* 38: 296–311.

Urban Appalachian Council. 1989. *Appalachian Idea Book*, Cincinnati: Cincinnati Public Schools.

Urban Environmental Conference. 1985. *Taking Back Our Health: An Institute on Surviving the Toxic Threat to Minority Communities.* Washington, DC: Urban Environment.

U.S. Environmental Protection Agency. 1992. "Environmental Equity: Reducing Risk for All Communities." *Workgroup Report to the Administrator*, Vol. 1. Washington, DC: author.

U.S. General Accounting Office. 1983. *Siting of Hazardous Waste Landfills and Their Correlation with Racial and Economic Status of Surrounding Communities.* Washington, DC: author.

Van Liere, Kent, and Riley E. Dunlap. 1980. "The Social Bases of Environmental Concern: A Review of Hypotheses, Explanations, and Empirical Evidence." *Public Opinion Quarterly* 44: 181–97.

Wagner, Thomas E. 1977. "Urban Schools and Appalachian Children." *Urban Education* 11 (3): 283–96.

——. 1987. "Introduction." In *Too Few Tomorrows: Urban Appalachians in the 1980s*, edited by Phillip J. Obermiller and William W. Philliber. Boone, NC: Appalachian Consortium Press.

Wahler, R. G., and W. H. Cormier. 1970. "The Ecological Interview: A First Step in Outpatient Child Behavior Therapy. *Journal of Behavior Therapy and Experimental Psychiatry* 1: 279–89.

Walls, David. 1976. "Appalachian Problems Are National Problems." *Appalachian Journal* 4 (1): 34–42.

——. 1978. "Internal Colony or Internal Periphery? A Critique of Current Models and an Alternative Formulation." In *Colonialism in Modern America: The Appalachian Case*, edited by Helen Lewis, Linda Johnson, and Don Askins. Boone, NC: Appalachian Consortium .

Watkins, H. V. M. 1973. "Consideration of Factors Relevant to the Development of Adequate Health Support Systems for Appalachian Migrants." Master's thesis, University of Cincinnati.

Watkins, Virginia McCoy, and Diana Gullett Trevino. 1982. "Occupational and Employment Status of Appalachian Migrant Women." In *Critical Essays in Appalachian Life and Culture*, edited by Richard Simon. Boone, NC: Appalachian Consortium.

Weiland, Steven, Thomas E. Wagner, and Phillip J. Obermiller, eds. 1978. *Perspectives on Urban Appalachians*. Cincinnati: Ohio Urban Appalachian Awareness Project, University of Cincinnati.

Weller, Jack. 1965. *Yesterday's People: Life in Contemporary Appalachia*. Lexington: University of Kentucky Press.

White, Stephen E. 1983. "Return Migration to Appalachian Kentucky: An Atypical Case of Nonmetropolitan Migration Reversal." *Rural Sociology* 48: 471–491.

Whitson, S. Mont, ed. 1988. *Sense of Place in Appalachia*. Morehead, KY: Office of Development Services, Morehead State University.

Wigginton, Eliot, ed. 1973. *Foxfire 2*. Garden City, NY: Anchor.

Willems, E. P. 1969. "Planning a Rationale for Naturalistic Research." In *Naturalistic Viewpoints in Psychological Research*, edited by E. P. Willems and H.L. Raush. New York: Holt, Rinehart, and Winston.

Willems, E. P., and H. L. Rausch, eds. 1969. *Naturalistic Viewpoints in Psychological Research*. New York: Holt, Rinehart, and Winston.

Zwerdling, Daniel. 1973. "Poverty and Pollution." *Progressive* 37: 25–29.

Index

About the Contributors

Barbara Baker is a graduate student in the College of Education at the University of Cincinnati.

Edwin C. Barnes is a faculty instructor in the Department of Medicine at the University of Cincinnati.

David Barnett is a professor in the College of Education at the University of Cincinnati.

Anne Bauer is an associate professor in the College of Education at the University of Cincinnati.

Kathryn M. Borman is a professor in the College of Education at the University of Cincinnati.

M. Kathryn Brown is a doctoral candidate in the Department of Biostatistics and Epidemiology at the University of Cincinnati.

Johanna S. DeStefano is a professor of Language and Literary Education at The Ohio State University.

Kristal E. Ehrhardt is a research associate in the College of Education at the University of Cincinnati.

Rhoda H. Halperin is a professor in the Department of Anthropology at the University of Cincinnati.

Walter S. Handy, Jr., is an assistant commissioner in the Cincinnati Health Department.

Lonnie R. Helton is an assistant professor in the Department of Social Work at Cleveland State University.

Fred Hoeweler is the youth employment coordinator at the Urban Appalachian Council in Cincinnati.

Michael E. Maloney is a social planner for the Appalachian People's Service Organization in Cincinnati.

Clyde B. McCoy is a professor in the School of Medicine at the University of Miami.

H. Virginia McCoy is an assistant professor in the Department of Public Health at Florida International University.

Phillip J. Obermiller is a research associate of the Appalachian Center at the University of Kentucky.

Robert W. Oldendick is director of The Institute of Public Affairs at the University of South Carolina.

Elizabeth M. Penn is an assistant professor in the Department of Education at Thomas More College.

Ray Rappold is a doctoral candidate in geography at the University of North Carolina at Chapel Hill.

Andrew Smith is a research associate in the Institute for Policy Research at the University of Cincinnati.

Delores Stegelin is an associate professor in the College of Education at the University of Cincinnati.

Stephanie Stollar is a doctoral candidate in the College of Education at the University of Cincinnati.

Diana Gullett Trevino is a teacher in the Cincinnati Public School System.